ATLAS OF

VASCULAR
SURGERY

Basic Techniques
and Exposures

ATLAS OF
VASCULAR SURGERY

Basic Techniques and Exposures

ROBERT B. RUTHERFORD, M.D.

Professor of Surgery
University of Colorado Health Sciences Center
Denver, Colorado

Illustrations by John Foerster
with Assistance from Tom McCracken

W.B. SAUNDERS COMPANY
A Division of Harcourt Brace & Company

Philadelphia   London   Toronto   Montreal   Sydney   Tokyo

W.B. SAUNDERS COMPANY
A Division of
Harcourt Brace & Company

The Curtis Center
Independence Square West
Philadelphia, Pennsylvania 19106

Library of Congress Cataloging-in-Publication Data

Rutherford, Robert B.

  Atlas of vascular surgery : basic techniques and exposures / Robert B. Rutherford : illustrations by John Foerster with assistance from Tom McCracken.

        p.   cm.

  Includes index.

  ISBN 0–7216–2956–3

  1. Blood-vessels—Surgery—Atlases.   I. Title.
  [DNLM: 1. Vascular Surgery—methods—atlases.
  WG 17 R975a]

  RD598.5.R88 1993

  617.4′13059—dc20

  DNLM/DLC   92–48878

ATLAS OF VASCULAR SURGERY:
BASIC TECHNIQUES AND EXPOSURES   ISBN 0–7216–2956–3

Printed in the United States of America

Last digit is the print number: 9   8   7   6   5   4

PREFACE

The author must confess to a long-standing disappointment in surgical atlases, particularly those in which the illustrations focus mostly on the final stages without demonstrating the essential intermediate steps. The proper positions, optional skin incisions, best routes through the underlying anatomy to gain proper exposure, and practical stepwise sequences for performing the procedure were often omitted or not well described. On the other hand, repetitiously depicting each technical aspect of every vascular procedure would be impractical and, ultimately, no more cost effective than atlases filled with beautiful but expensive color illustrations.

This atlas of vascular surgery "grew" out of attempts to describe the basic and essential techniques involved in performing vascular surgical procedures in an organized and usable format for the training of surgical residents. It was originally conceived to be no more than a simple "primer" on vascular surgery technique or, at best, an illustrated manual. Once the idea of adding *vascular exposures* to *basic vascular techniques,* as the two essential technical foundations of vascular surgery, was entertained, it was a natural extension to then combine them into one volume first with descriptions of specific operations to be presented later in a second volume. This would avoid repeating all the similar details of exposure and basic technique, focusing on the essential differences such as patient positioning, extent of the sterile field, choice of the incision and exposure, creation of the proper connecting anatomic pathways or "tunnels," choice of graft, and correct sequence of performing the component steps of the operation.

Thus, this project has grown, in stages, into a full and complete atlas. Its development is reflected in its organization into basic vascular techniques, common vascular exposures, and finally individual vascular operations. Obviously, many worthwhile technical variations exist other than those featured in this single-author work. These particular techniques and maneuvers have evolved over 25 years of applying and modifying those originally learned during training that now serve the author well. It is hoped that they will provide a useful framework upon which young surgeons may build and will offer alternative techniques for established surgeons to consider incorporating into their armamentarium.

CONTENTS____

BASIC VASCULAR TECHNIQUES

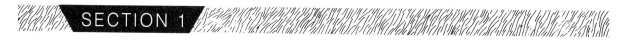
Basic Vascular Techniques

This first section focuses on the basic vascular techniques that are common to many procedures—e.g., dissection, exposure, isolation, and control of vessels; intraoperative hemostasis and anticoagulation; vascular incisions and closures; and basic anastomotic techniques. The basic principles of the bypass graft, interposition graft, and endoaneurysmal reconstruction are also illustrated. Certain other common procedures are included: thromboembolectomy, endarterectomy, "vein harvest," vein valvulotomy (as used in the in situ technique), tunneling for the passage of a graft between two incisions, and completion angiography.

HISTORICAL BACKGROUND

The first recorded vascular reconstruction was reported by Lambert in 1762. He described Hallowell's closure, in 1759, of a small opening in a brachial artery, performed with a pin around which a thread was twisted. This was a historic step because, prior to that time, restoration of flow had always been sacrificed for the sake of hemostasis, and vessel ligation was essentially the only vascular procedure practiced. Unfortunately, Asman's subsequent failure to achieve patency following vascular repair, using similar techniques in experimental animals, discouraged the surgeons of the day, and for almost a century thereafter it was believed that suture material entering the lumen of a vessel invariably would produce an obliterating thrombosis.

By 1882, Schede had accomplished the first successful lateral vein repair. The first direct vascular anastomosis was probably Nikolai Eck's lateral anastomosis, in 1877, between the inferior vena cava and the portal vein of dogs. In this innovative technique, the opposing surfaces of the two vessels were sutured together by two parallel rows of interrupted sutures. A suture at one corner was temporarily left untied so that a special instrument could be inserted to slit open each vessel in order to allow cross-flow through the anastomosis. Although this was technically a lateral, or side-to-side, anastomosis, it was then converted to an end-to-side portacaval shunt by ligating the hepatic limb of the portal vein. It is interesting to reflect on Eck's enduring fame as a result of this experiment, considering that he had only one survivor and produced no other significant contributions to surgery.

In 1899, Kümmell performed the first end-to-end anastomosis of an artery in a human, if one discounts Murphy's "mechanical button" invagination anastomosis

2 years earlier. As a background to these and other sporadic clinical successes, the decades surrounding the turn of this century witnessed numerous experimental studies evaluating almost every conceivable suture technique. Absorbable versus nonabsorbable suture and continuous versus interrupted, simple versus mattress, and everting versus edge-to-edge approximation techniques all were tried. These endeavors culminated in the classic studies of Carrel and Guthrie, which firmly established the basic principles and techniques of modern vascular anastomosis prior to World War I. These investigators were also the first to achieve significant experimental success with fresh and preserved homografts and heterografts for vascular replacement and bypass. When, in 1906, Goyanes used a segment of popliteal vein to bridge a defect caused by the excision of an aneurysm of the accompanying artery and, the next year, Lexer used the saphenous vein for arterial reconstruction following excision of an axillary artery aneurysm, the stage appeared to be set for vascular surgery to enter the modern era. However, in spite of continuing, though sporadic, reports of other clinical successes such as these, widespread application of these principles and techniques did not occur for almost 40 years. The reasons for this delay are not entirely clear, but the development of better diagnostic techniques, especially angiography, the evolution of vascular prostheses and homograft storage methods, the development of techniques that allowed thoracotomy to be performed at reasonable risk, plus the availability of heparin and type-specific, cross-matched blood, all appear to have been important in the final launching of the "golden era of cardiovascular surgery," which began just *after* World War II.

Before the technical explosion that followed in the 1950s, arterial ligation for vascular trauma, arteriovenous fistulas, or aneurysms; simple vascular repair with or without local thrombectomy for acute occlusion; sympathectomy for chronic ischemia; and a variety of amputations were the mainstays of surgery for peripheral arterial disease. The introduction first of arterial homografts and then of a succession of plastic prostheses culminating in the array of knitted and woven Dacron grafts available today; the emerging preference for fresh venous and arterial autografts for smaller arterial replacement, along with the development of in situ techniques; and, finally, the additional availability of the human umbilical vein allograft and the expanded polytetrafluoroethylene (PTFE) graft have provided the vascular surgeon with an adequate array of arterial substitutes for most situations. Unfortunately, the concomitant development and refinement of vascular suture materials, atraumatic vascular clamps, and other mechanical devices such as vena caval clips and embolectomy catheters have received almost better coverage in manufacturers' brochures than in formal surgical literature.

INSTRUMENTS AND SUTURE MATERIAL

The *basic* instruments required for simple vascular procedures are not very different from the standard instruments used in any operative dissection, essentially including only vascular forceps, a fine-pointed diamond-jawed needle holder, a right-angle clamp, and scissors for dissecting and opening vessels (Fig. 1). During maneuvers to dissect, free, and encircle vessels, a right-angle clamp with fine (but not too pointed) tips is invaluable. Different sizes of Metzenbaum scissors are ideal for dissection on or around the vessels because they do *not* have sharp-pointed tips and are less likely to injure the vessel inadvertently. On the other hand, because they *do* have delicately pointed tips, straight, curved, or angled Potts scissors are preferable for incising or excising the vessel wall itself, once it has been opened with a No. 11 scalpel blade.

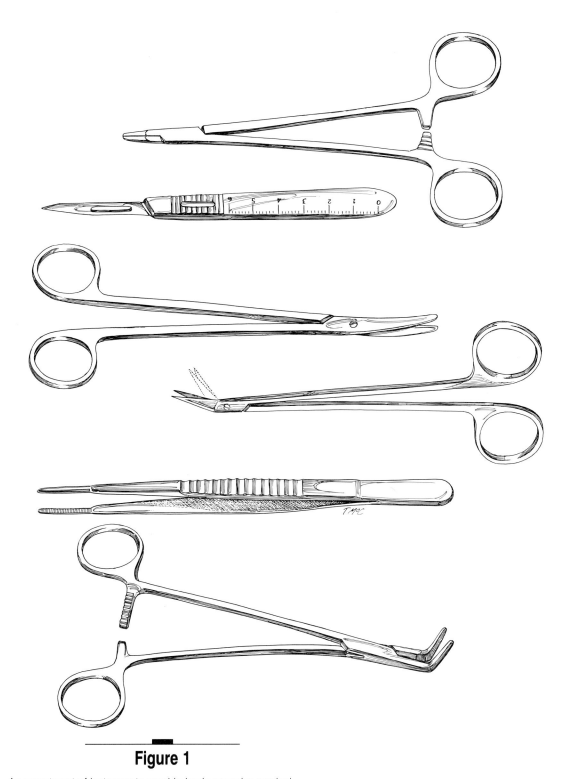

Figure 1

An assortment of instruments used in basic vascular surgical procedures. From top to bottom, a slender-tipped, diamond-jawed needle holder, a No. 11 scalpel blade (for initiating arteriotomy), blunt-tipped Metzenbaum scissors to dissect vessels and variously angled Potts scissors to open them, fine tissue grasping forceps, and a right-angle clamp to create a passage around vessels so they may be encircled with tapes.

Basic Vascular Techniques

An assortment of atraumatic vascular clamps is also required (Fig. 2). The different sizes and shapes of vascular clamps are necessary to accommodate differences in degree of exposure, depth of wound, size of vessel, and angle of application (i.e., transverse, oblique, or tangential). Vascular clamps usually have fine teeth or serrations that are offset and interdigitating, allowing them to grip and occlude the vessel wall without crushing or slipping, as exemplified by the jaws of the DeBakey clamps shown in Figure 3 (top). Fogarty has developed a Hydragrip clamp, with straight or angled configuration, into the jaws of which a variety of soft "flat," "toothed," or "bristled" plastic inserts may be placed. The jaws of these are shown in Figure 3 (bottom). They are particularly useful in clamping PTFE grafts during arterial reconstruction.

In addition to these vascular clamps, with handles that allow them to be held and with which vessel position can be manipulated, there are smaller vascular clamps without handles, the jaws of which are held in the occlusive position by a springlike mechanism. These include the standard bulldog clamps, the Gregory and Fogarty bulldog clamps, and the larger-sized neurosurgical aneurysm or Heifitz clips shown in Figure 4. They are useful when working on smaller vessels or in controlling branches or tributaries, particularly when the exposure is limited. Most of the older-design bulldog clamps are too traumatic because pressure cannot be easily controlled at lesser levels. The Gregory long-handled bulldog and the Fogarty spring bulldog clamps are much better in this regard and are useful when they can be accommodated within the dimensions of the wound. For smaller collateral branches, particularly when exposure is limited, a thin-bladed Heifitz clip, employed by neurosurgeons to occlude intracranial vessels (e.g., in berry aneurysm surgery), may also be useful.

Moistened umbilical tapes, thin rubber catheters, or Silastic loops are used to encircle major vessels and their large branches or tributaries during dissection and manipulation. A heavy silk suture, doubly looped around a small branch or tributary, can, by the weight of a hemostat clamped to its end, control intraoperative bleeding from these branches without crowding the operative field with additional vascular clamps. Finally, as illustrated later, balloon catheters are useful for occluding vessels as well as removing intravascular thrombus.

Microvascular surgery is not covered in this text. Performed under an operating microscope, it uses instruments and techniques that are quite different from those just described. On the other hand, most of today's vascular surgeons are quite adept at carrying out the *same* basic techniques illustrated in the pages that follow, on quite small (1 to 2 mm in diameter) vessels (e.g., radial, ulnar, dorsalis pedis, posterior tibial, and lateral plantar arteries) using $2\times$ to $3\times$ loupe magnification. Here, in what might be called "minivascular surgery," the techniques are similar to those of standard vascular procedures but some microvascular instruments are used such as small Beaver blades, jeweler's forceps, and Castroviejo needle holders and scissors, as shown in Figure 5.

The selection of vascular suture material, like that of vascular instruments, is to some extent an individual matter, and every surgeon has favorites. The caliber of the suture should be as fine as possible, short of risking suture line disruption and anastomotic aneurysm formation, to minimize hemorrhage through suture holes and the amount of suture material in contact with the vessel lumen. As a frame of reference, a range from 2-0 to 8-0 is used in most clinical practice, as the surgeon progresses from the aorta centrally to the wrist or crural arteries peripherally. For the most common peripheral anastomoses, e.g., in femoropopliteal bypass, 5-0 or 6-0 sutures usually are preferred, whereas 2-0 and 3-0 are preferred for the aorta; 4-0, the iliacs; and 7-0 or 8-0, the small tibial anastomoses.

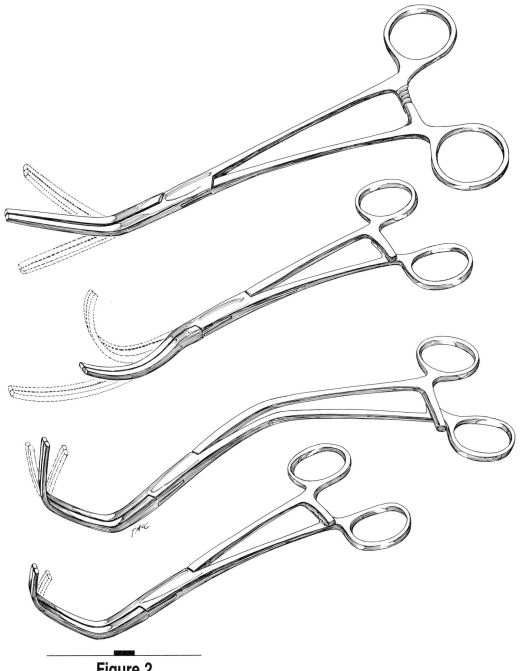

Figure 2

An assortment of differently shaped atraumatic vascular clamps.
From top to bottom, straight and angled clamps, spoon-shaped
or other curved configurations, and Satinsky-shaped clamps with
various handles and jaw angles and lengths. (The Satinsky clamp
was originally designed to control the tip of an atrial appendage
while a purse-string suture was placed and was used to enter
and withdraw from that chamber, but, with the addition of
interdigitating serrated teeth and a variety of sizes, it has become
one of the most versatile clamps for peripheral vascular
procedures.)

Basic Vascular Techniques

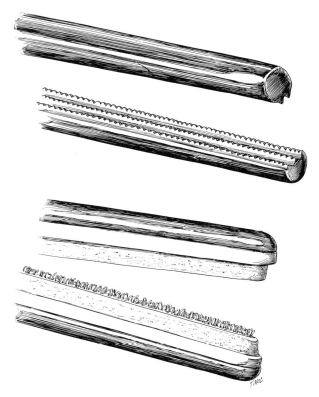

Figure 3

Top, The basic design of serrated rows of interdigitating teeth, which characterizes the DeBakey-type vascular clamps so prevalent in current practice. *Bottom,* The soft Hydragrip vascular clamps designed by Fogarty come with an assortment of disposable inserts that snap into place on the inside of the metal jaws. Shown here are the plain surface (above) and the bristled surface (below), the latter offering resistance to side slippage.

All vascular sutures should be swaged onto fine, one-half or three-eighths circle, round needles with tapered or beveled tips. Flattening the body of such a fine needle parallel to the radius of its curve and placing a tapered cutting edge on the side of its tip facilitate penetration through hard arteriosclerotic plaques and avoid bending the body of the needle during penetration. The metal composition of vascular needles has been steadily improved from stainless steel through a number of alloys that resist deforming even in the most delicate sizes and configurations, although heavily calcified vessels, more commonly seen in diabetic or chronic renal failure patients, still present difficulties. Braided silk, lubricated with sterile mineral oil or bone wax, handles well and is still satisfactory for venous anastomoses, but monofilament polypropylene is now usually preferred for arterial (and venous) work because of greater strength and durability and reduced tissue reactivity. The latter is the author's preference in most instances, although the handling properties of the new Gore-Tex suture make it most attractive. It is now routine practice to use the double swaged-on vascular suture (i.e., with a needle on each end) to allow more flexibility and speed in performing vascular anastomoses.

Much has been made of the larger caliber of the needle relative to the suture in producing holes in vessels and grafts (particularly thin-walled PTFE prostheses), producing persistent, troublesome bleeding. Although the author applauds efforts to combat this diameter mismatch (with use of smaller laser-drilled needle holes to hold the suture and suture that expands beyond its attachment to match more closely the caliber of the needle), much of this problem relates to the surgeon's technique of needle placement and passage. Always penetrating the vessel-graft wall at 90°, faithfully following the curve of the needle during the entire needle passage, and pronating another 180° at the wrist between needle insertion and needle withdrawal to allow the latter to occur more smoothly will eliminate unnecessarily large needle holes, most of which are due to iatrogenic tears rather than needles that are too large.

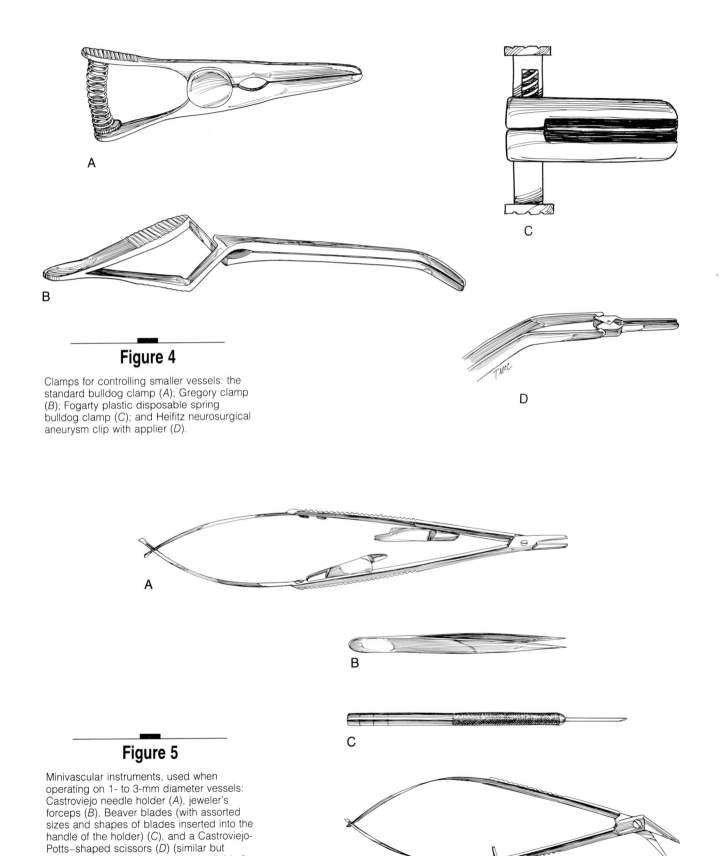

Figure 4

Clamps for controlling smaller vessels: the
standard bulldog clamp (*A*); Gregory clamp
(*B*); Fogarty plastic disposable spring
bulldog clamp (*C*); and Heifitz neurosurgical
aneurysm clip with applier (*D*).

Figure 5

Minivascular instruments, used when
operating on 1- to 3-mm diameter vessels:
Castroviejo needle holder (*A*), jeweler's
forceps (*B*), Beaver blades (with assorted
sizes and shapes of blades inserted into the
handle of the holder) (*C*), and a Castroviejo-
Potts–shaped scissors (*D*) (similar but
curved-tipped scissors are also available for
dissecting vessels).

VASCULAR EXPOSURE AND CONTROL

Vascular exposure and control are usually the first orders of business during any vascular operation. They are usually completed *before* systemic heparinization to minimize blood loss and maintain a "dry" field to facilitate preliminary dissection. The particular approaches employed in exploring and exposing specific vascular segments are covered in detail in Section 2, but the principles of exposure are discussed here. A close familiarity with the anatomic relationships of the vascular segment to be exposed, including the topical anatomy governing the location and length of the incision, is essential. In most cases, the incision is made longitudinally over the course of the vessel, extending a few centimeters at each end beyond the required length of exposed vessel, unless the vessel is deeply placed, in which case considerable additional length of incision is required. One cannot always expect to be guided by the underlying pulse in placing the incision because, by the very nature of the problem at hand, the vessel may often be occluded or at least pulseless beyond an obstruction. Furthermore, even if pulsatile, many arterial segments are too deep to be palpated easily with the gloved finger. Thus, knowledge of topical anatomy and employing reliable landmarks are essential in making the correct incision. This is clearly illustrated in Section 2.

After incising the skin, passing through the overlying subcutaneous fat and fascia, and retracting intervening muscles to the side, the vessels are finally approached. They are usually surrounded by a variable amount of fatty tissue and often enveloped in a sheath so they do not simply appear "naked" as they do in anatomy books and surgical atlases. At this point in the dissection even a weak pulse can be palpated in many vessels to guide the dissection. If there is no pulse, the occluded vessel, especially if calcified, is often readily palpated and rolled as a firm cord running longitudinally under the exploring finger. In difficult dissections, typified by reoperation through scar tissue, there may be no tactile clues. A sterile Doppler probe may be helpful, outlining the course of an artery with its postobstructive flow signals or at least the location of the major adjacent vein, in which the relationship with the artery is known. Collaterals may be confusing if one does not attempt to follow the longitudinal course of the main vessel with the Doppler probe. Collateral vessels almost never run a straight course for any significant distance.

In dissecting out the artery, it is important to stay in a plane as close to the outer adventitia as possible. The artery may have an additional investiture of connective tissue in addition to the formal sheath that one may find surrounding many vessels (e.g., the proximal femoral vessels). If there is an inflammatory reaction around the artery, commonly seen to some extent in those involved by the atherosclerotic process and invariably in those with true inflammatory disease (e.g., nonspecific aortoarteritis and thromboangiitis obliterans), it is common for inexperienced surgeons to dissect too far away from the artery, well outside the adventitial plane. It is best to dissect *closer* to the artery until one finds the telltale adventitial surface with its characteristic vasovasorum pattern. Staying a "safe distance" away from the vessel surface is actually *not* safer; the safest plane is as close to the vessel surface as possible. Once one has reached this correct plane, it is usually easy to continue to follow it along, because it can be readily recognized by what some have called the "adventitial white line." This plane immediately adjacent to the adventitial surface appears to whiten when countertraction is applied perpendicularly to it and air is drawn into the intervening areolar tissue. Thus, with traction and countertraction on the vessel and the surrounding tissues to bring out this white line and gently dissecting along it with the blunt end of Metzenbaum scissors, an adequate segment of the artery is usually readily exposed (Fig. 6). Ordinarily, nothing crosses this periadventitial plane other than collateral branches and, by staying in it, one not only can easily identify these branches as they appear but also can avoid injury to surrounding structures and minimize bleeding from small vessels in the area. Many arteries, typified by the popliteal and tibial arteries, are surrounded by a network of small but annoying venae comitantes. Again, by staying close to the artery, in this areolar plane, only those venae comitantes crossing directly in front of the line of dissection need to be dealt with.

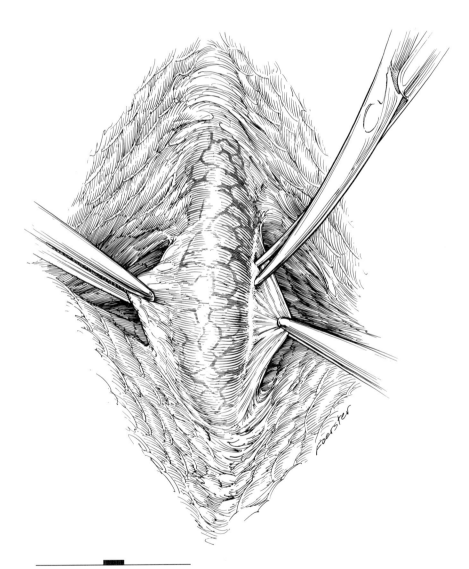

Figure 6

Dissecting out a normal artery, with its characteristic vasa vasorum, is facilitated by perpendicular countertraction, which draws air into the periadventitial areolar tissue and creates a white line that identifies the correct plane.

Basic Vascular Techniques

Reoperations on vessels surrounded by dense scar tissue present special difficulties in dissection because the characteristic adventitial markings that identify arterial segments and the surrounding loose areolar tissue that provides an easy entry plane are obscured and the blunt-tipped Metzenbaum scissors do not readily cut through scar tissue. Here, keeping in mind the usual longitudinal orientation of the main vessels and using lateral traction perpendicular to this, it is usually possible to identify favorable dissection planes to enter. Even with a heavy investiture of scar tissue, arteries usually maintain a thin layer of periadventitial areolar tissue around them and countertracture will still reveal this as a fine white line. If the Metzenbaum scissors will not readily dissect in this plane, a scalpel blade, held more perpendicularly like a pen but with the blade oriented at almost 90° to the line of dissection, can be stroked along this white line parallel to the adjacent artery (Fig. 7). Once the correct feel of the obliquely angled cutting edge of the scalpel blade has been mastered, this will usually become the preferred method of dissection in difficult "redo" operations.

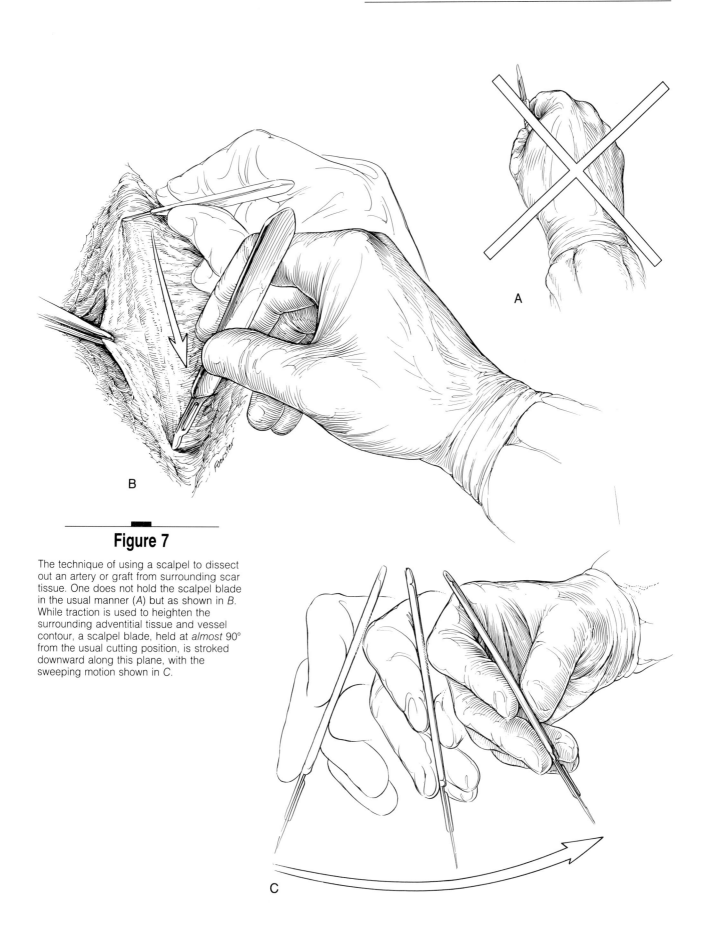

Figure 7

The technique of using a scalpel to dissect
out an artery or graft from surrounding scar
tissue. One does not hold the scalpel blade
in the usual manner (A) but as shown in B.
While traction is used to heighten the
surrounding adventitial tissue and vessel
contour, a scalpel blade, held at *almost* 90°
from the usual cutting position, is stroked
downward along this plane, with the
sweeping motion shown in C.

Basic Vascular Techniques

In most operations, it is best to begin directly by dissecting out the artery in the middle of the field and encircling it with a moistened umbilical tape, using a right-angle clamp passed carefully through an opening dissected under the artery (Fig. 8A). Traction on this will draw the artery up and away from the surrounding structures and put its major and collateral branches on a stretch, which makes them easier to detect as the dissection proceeds proximally and distally (Fig. 8B). *The principle of using traction and countertraction to aid in the dissection of major arteries cannot be overemphasized.* It not only delineates the proper adventitial plane of dissection, even in scarred reoperative cases, but it also draws the artery away from the surrounding structures (which might otherwise be inadvertently injured) and helps identify collateral branches and crossing veins before they are unintentionally divided.

Once the desired length of the arterial segment has been exposed, it must be controlled (i.e., occluded proximally and distally) with atraumatic devices, before opening. For this purpose, the umbilical tape, used initially for traction, is usually slid upward to the proximal end and Silastic tapes are *doubly* looped around the distal end of the segment and any major branches. By pulling on this double "Potts loop," the vessel may be atraumatically occluded without the need to apply a clamp (Fig. 9). Usually a vascular clamp rather than a Silastic tape is applied proximally because it provides more secure control, but the umbilical tape is left in place to facilitate application and reapplication of the proximal clamp during flushing maneuvers (Fig. 10). A second doubly looped Silastic tape at the upper end, rather than an umbilical tape and vascular clamp, is an acceptable means of obtaining proximal control when dealing with smaller peripheral arterial segments. However, when two Silastic tapes are drawn strongly in opposite directions, they often tend to pull the arteriotomy too tightly shut, preventing ready access for intraluminal procedures, closure, or anastomosis (Fig. 11A). Furthermore, if temporarily loosened, or if traction is applied in an upward or lateral direction, these loops tend to slide centrally and may ultimately crowd the arteriotomy (Fig. 11B). The latter problem can be obviated if the double loop straddles a distal branch, not only controlling the latter but also preventing the slick Silastic tape from sliding up or down (Fig. 11C and D).

Placing straight vascular clamps perpendicularly on the arterial segment above and below the intended arteriotomy site has two potential disadvantages, shown in Figure 12A: the clamps may be unstable and shift back and forth, and they may, by rising straight up out of the wound, impede access with other instruments needed to carry out the intended procedure. Angled clamps can sometimes obviate this (Fig. 12B), if the wound edges are not too high. Figure 12C and D shows a method of *proximal* clamp application the author has used to avoid these problems. One jaw of a small Satinsky-shaped vascular clamp is placed under the proximal artery, approaching it from below and sliding it up as high as possible. By also laying it down flat against the wound edges before closing it, the clamp stays out of the surgeon's way.

The introduction of Silastic tapes was welcomed with great enthusiasm as a way of avoiding the need for applying vascular clamps, which, in spite of their "atraumatic" interdigitating teeth, are quite capable of injuring arteries—particularly diseased arteries in which there is considerable plaque or heavy mural calcification. Such injury can ultimately lead to fibrotic stenosis or clamp strictures. However, pulling too tightly on the doubled Silastic loop can also produce injury and the same undesirable end result—an arterial stricture. Typically, the two ends of the doubled Silastic loop are pulled up too tightly and clamped to the

Text continued on page 20

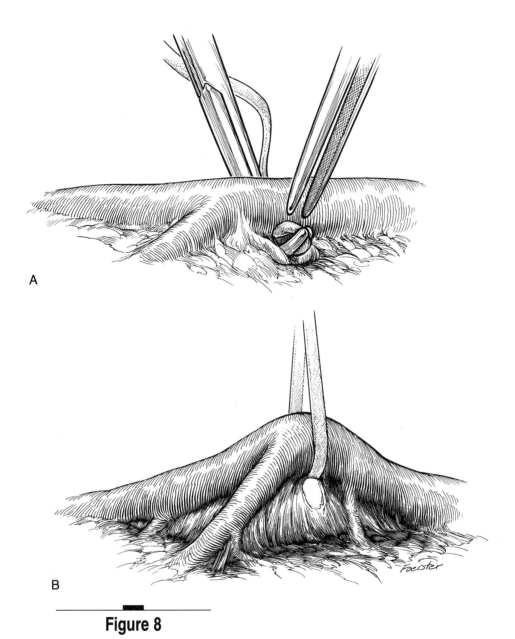

Figure 8

Dissection of an arterial segment is
facilitated by passing an umbilical tape
under it (*A*) because traction on this will
facilitate further dissection and reveal the
position of significant branches (*B*).

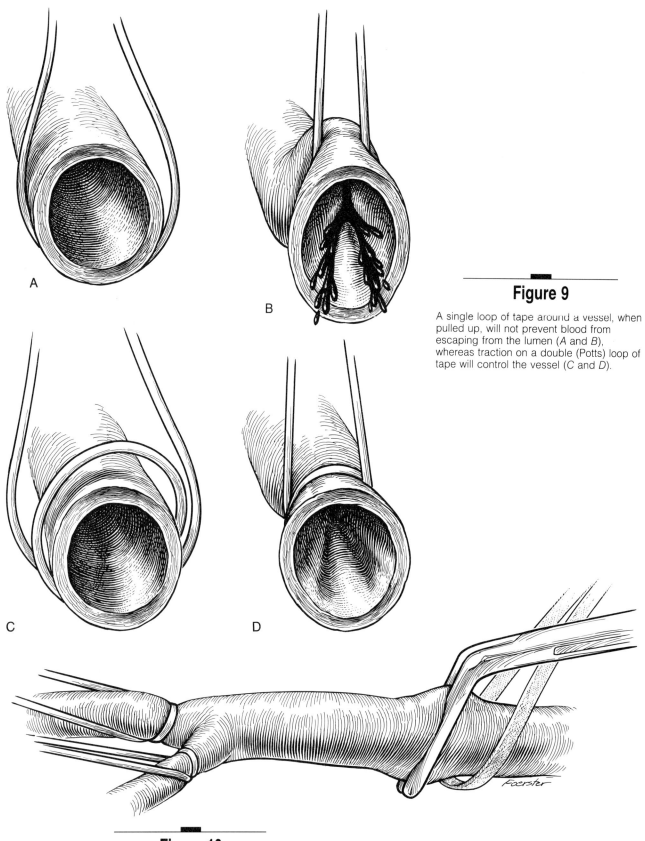

Figure 9

A single loop of tape around a vessel, when pulled up, will not prevent blood from escaping from the lumen (A and B), whereas traction on a double (Potts) loop of tape will control the vessel (C and D).

A

B

C

D

Figure 10

Double-looped tapes control the distal branches of the arterial segment, but a vascular clamp is preferred proximally to provide more secure occlusion without tension. The proximal umbilical tape is retained to facilitate clamp application and release during flushing maneuvers.

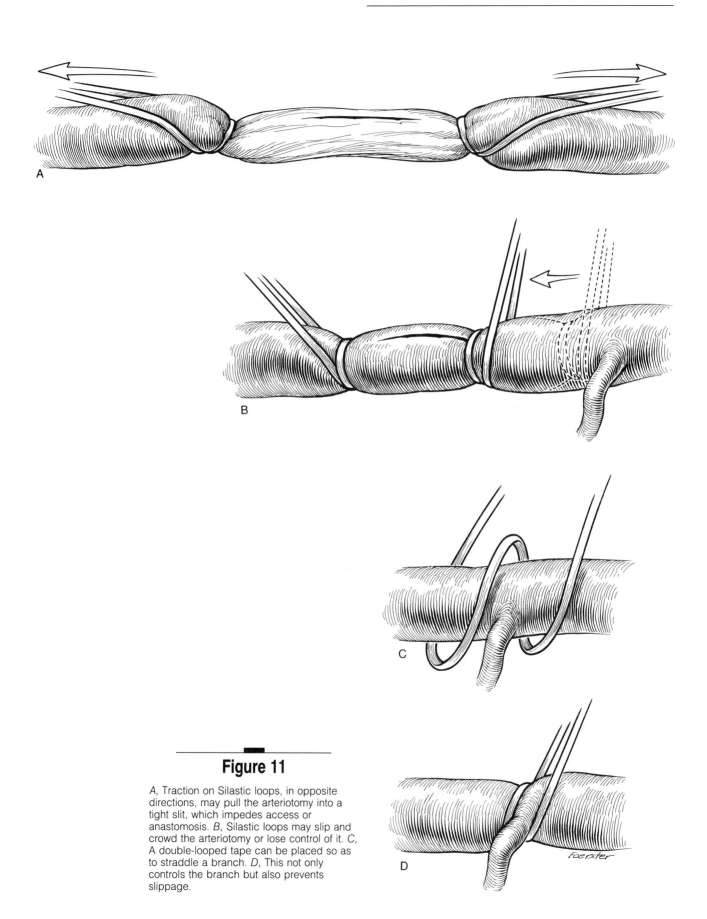

Figure 11

A, Traction on Silastic loops, in opposite directions, may pull the arteriotomy into a tight slit, which impedes access or anastomosis. *B,* Silastic loops may slip and crowd the arteriotomy or lose control of it. *C,* A double-looped tape can be placed so as to straddle a branch. *D,* This not only controls the branch but also prevents slippage.

Basic Vascular Techniques

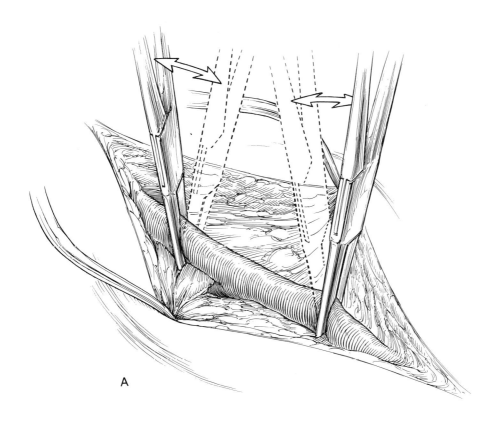

A

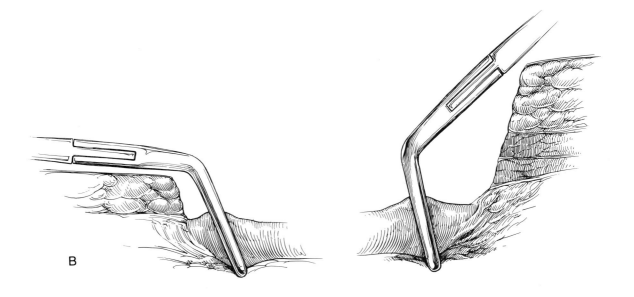

B

Figure 12

A, Perpendicularly applied straight vascular clamps can get in the way of the procedure and must be held to avoid shifting. B, Angled clamps can minimize this problem if their configuration conforms to the dimensions of the wound edges.

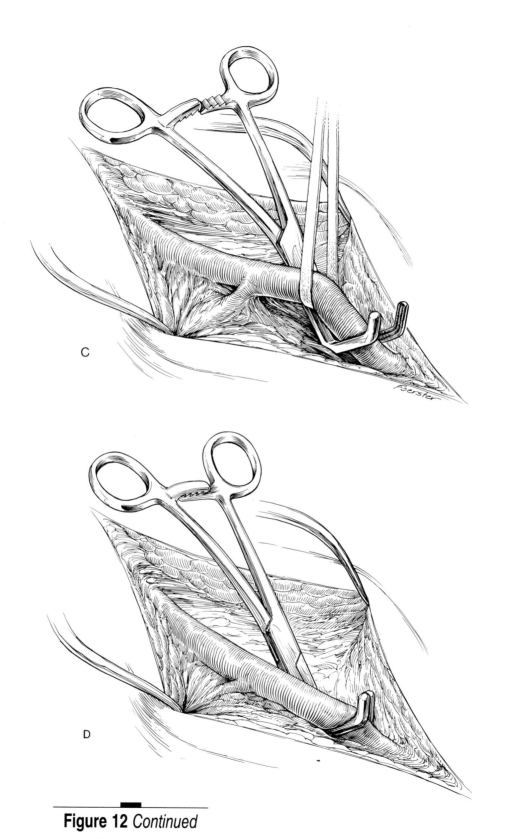

C

D

Figure 12 *Continued*

C and *D,* A method of applying a small
Satinsky-shaped vascular clamp that
provides unobtrusive proximal control.

Basic Vascular Techniques

surrounding drapes under too much tension, and usually the tension is not rechecked after the arteriotomy is made. The author prefers to bring the ends of each loop through the circular finger openings on the handles of the self-retaining retractors (e.g., Weitlaner or Gelpi), adjusting them just tight enough to stop bleeding, as visualized through the open arteriotomy, and then securing them in this position by cross-clamping them with the proximal jaw rather than the tip of the clamp. This way the protruding tips of the clamp project well beyond the Silastic loop, and thus they engage the circumference of the handle openings and cannot slip forward and through them (Fig. 13).

The foregoing methods of vascular control, by clamp or vessel loop, will suffice in the majority of circumstances, but a few other techniques with special application are mentioned here for the sake of completeness. The first is the use of a Rumel tourniquet. Here, a moistened umbilical tape is passed around the

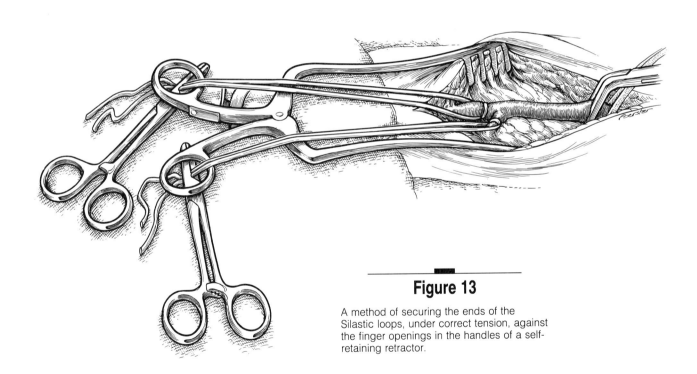

Figure 13

A method of securing the ends of the Silastic loops, under correct tension, against the finger openings in the handles of a self-retaining retractor.

artery and its ends are hooked by the Rumel instrument, which looks like a flat metal crochet hook over which a short segment of red rubber or plastic catheter has been passed (Fig. 14*A*). After the ends of the tape are pulled through the red rubber catheter (Fig. 14*B*), the artery can be occluded by downward pressure on the catheter, secured by application of a clamp (Fig. 14*C*). This allows repeated release and reocclusion and is particularly useful when inserting indwelling vascular shunts but, unless applied gently, can also cause vessel injury. Furthermore, it is not a secure method of controlling heavily calcified vessels. This can be a difficult problem, especially when dealing with the calcified tibial arteries commonly encountered in patients with diabetes. A sterile pneumatic tourniquet applied above the knee, as promulgated by Bernhard and Towne, avoids the need for direct application of occluding devices and even dissecting out and encircling the vessels.

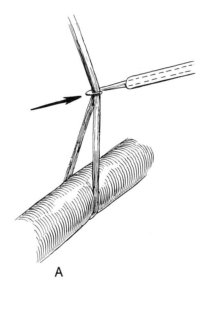

A

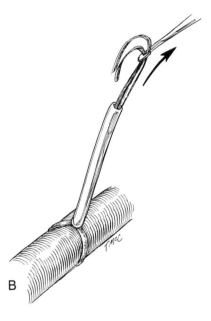

B

Figure 14

Application of a Rumel tourniquet. *A,* Hooking the two ends of the umbilical tape; *B,* pulling the tape ends through the short segment of rubber catheter; and *C,* cinching down the tourniquet and securing it with a hemostat.

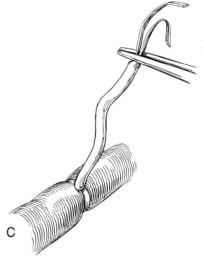

C

Basic Vascular Techniques

Circumferential control of the aorta and iliac arteries may be difficult, when performed in the usual fashion, because of the limited exposure and the lumbar arteries or iliac veins, respectively, located on their posterior aspect. One approach that works well on the infrarenal aorta involves passage of a renal pedicle clamp through a small posterior opening and drawing the tip of a red rubber catheter back around the aorta (Fig. 15*A*). This maneuver provides an advantage over the usual umbilical tape in that the lower jaw of a curved or an angled (e.g., Satinsky) vascular clamp can be pushed into the flanged end of the catheter and *drawn* into position under the aorta, without risk of injuring lumbar arteries or the vena cava

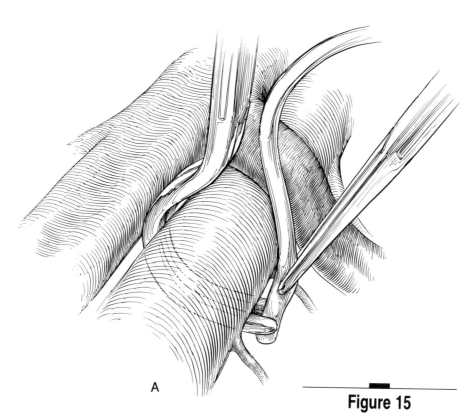

A

Figure 15

By passage of a flanged red rubber catheter (12 to 14F) around the infrarenal aorta (*A*), the tip of a vascular clamp can be inserted snugly in the flange and drawn into position by catheter traction without inadvertently injuring lumbar arteries or the inferior vena cava (*B*). The clamp is closed without removing the catheter, which is left in place for subsequent maneuvers (*C*).

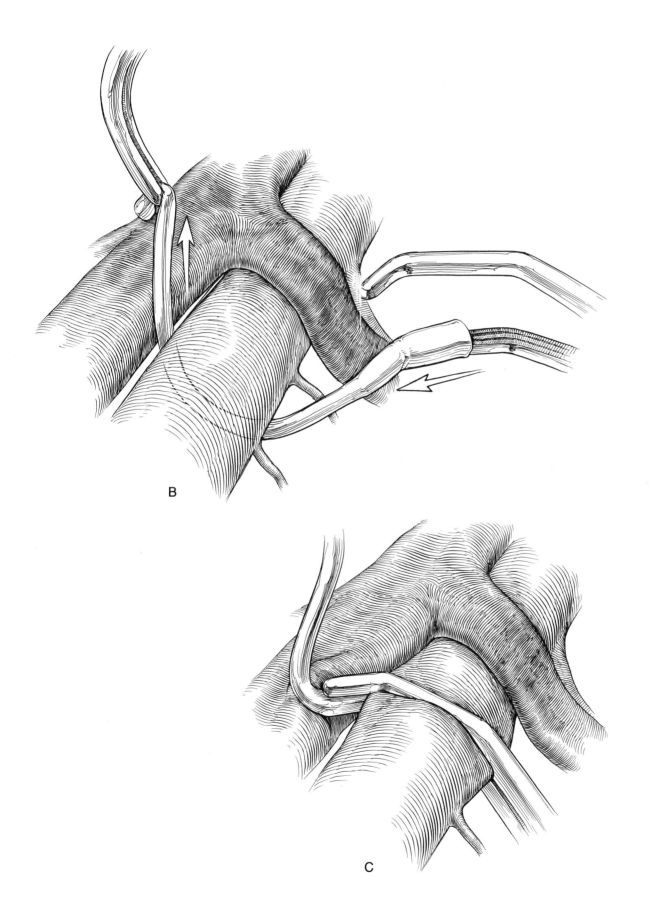

B

C

Basic Vascular Techniques

(Fig. 15*B* and *C*). However, aortic encirclement is often unnecessary and cannot be done quickly in emergency situations. Thus, in most instances, clamps are simply applied vertically, with each jaw inserted into an opening on either side of the aorta and slid down until they abut the vertebral body, and then they are closed (Fig. 16). The "subtraction" method of encircling major deep branches, such as the internal iliac or profunda femoris anterior, is illustrated under iliac artery exposure (see Fig. 91).

PERMANENT VASCULAR INTERRUPTION

It may be necessary to interrupt flow through a vessel for a number of reasons—for example, ligation of a vein to prevent reflux (as in high ligation of the saphenous vein or perforator ligation), closure or control of arteriovenous fistulas, and arterial interruption to control inaccessible hemorrhage following trauma. Ordinarily, for *veins or smaller arteries* once an adequate segment has been exposed, single or double ligation in continuity with a large nonabsorbable ligature will suffice (Fig. 17*A* and *B*). If there is a possibility of recanalization, double ligation with an intervening transfixion suture, which penetrates the lumen, is the most secure method of ligation in continuity (Fig. 17*C*). If it is deemed necessary to divide the vessel, either large terminal ends ("cuffs") should be left beyond each ligature, which is suitable for small veins or arteries (Fig. 17*D*), or, for larger vessels, an additional suture ligature or metal clip can be placed beyond each of the initial ligatures for added security, so that they cannot be pushed off by the force of arterial pulsations (Fig. 17*E*).

Divided major arteries (e.g., greater than 6 mm in diameter) are best closed by a running, end-on suture, with at least the proximal or pulsatile end reinforced with an additional heavy proximal ligature (Fig. 18*A* and *B*). A colorful part of the early history of cardiovascular surgery focused on determining the best method of interrupting flow through a patent ductus arteriosus. Often this structure was large and short, with insufficient room for double-clamping, division, and end-on closure of each stump. In such a case, double heavy ligatures were placed at either end with a transfixion suture between them, thus obliterating the lumen so that it could be safely left in continuity, as previously shown in Figure 17*C*. When the ductus was broad and/or long enough, it was usually divided between vascular clamps and then oversewn, with or without a protecting ligature, as shown in Figure 18*A* and *B*. However, when removal of an infected graft is the indication for arterial interruption, monofilament, nonabsorbable (i.e., polypropylene) suture should be used to close the end of the artery *after* resection back to normal-appearing vessel (preferably confirmed first by frozen section histology and later by culture of the cut end). In the case of infection involving the aorta, a second proximal row of interrupted mattress sutures, rather than a simple reinforcing ligature, is recommended if room allows (Fig. 18*C*). Alternatively, a protective row of staples may be placed (Fig. 18*D*) if the aorta is *not* too heavily involved with calcified plaque. (Stapling heavily calcified aortas often leads to serious bleeding.) The intent here is to set up a protective barrier, applied from outside the lumen to isolate the stump closure, knowing that blowout of an infected aortic stump, closed in a single layer, is a well-recognized possibility in such situations.

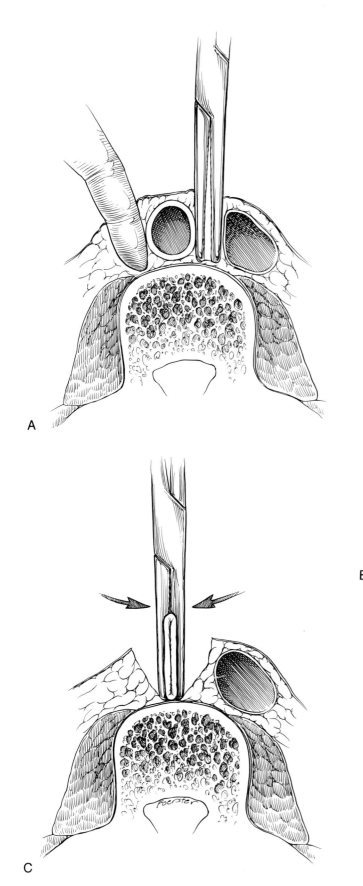

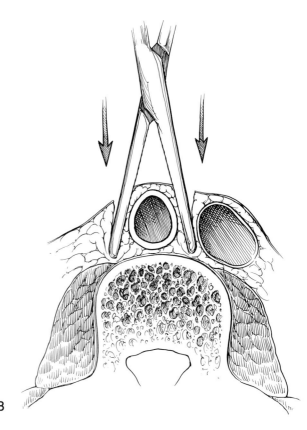

Figure 16

Once small finger openings are created on both sides of the aorta (*A*), the jaws of a vascular clamp can be vertically lowered into them on both sides (*B*), until they abut the vertebral bodies. Close the clamp to achieve aortic control (*C*).

Basic Vascular Techniques

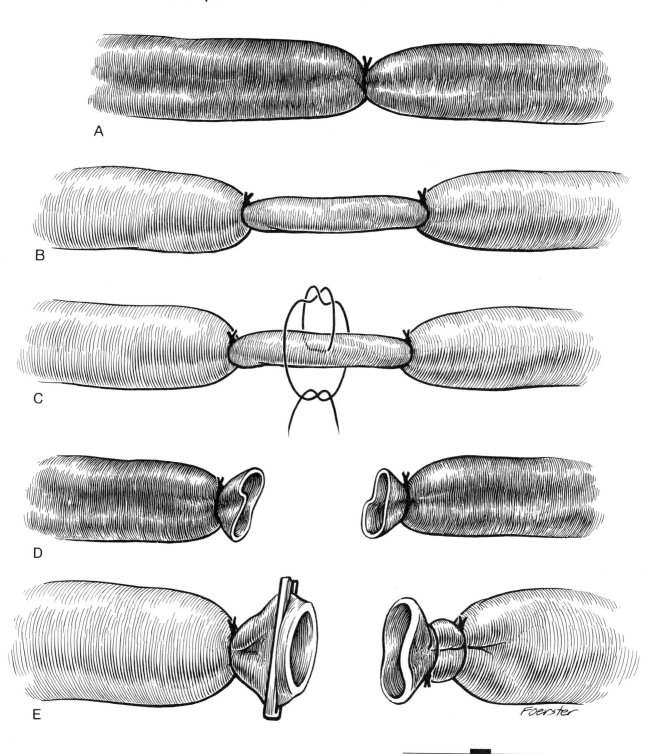

Figure 17

Vascular interruption techniques for small arteries and veins: *A,* Single ligation; *B,* double ligation in continuity; *C,* double ligation with intervening transfixion suture; *D,* double ligation and division; *E,* reinforcing ligatured ends with a transfixion suture or metal clip.

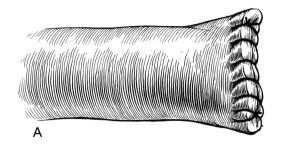

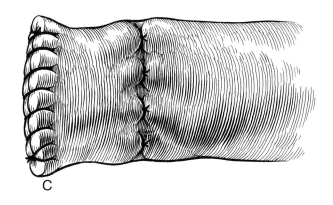

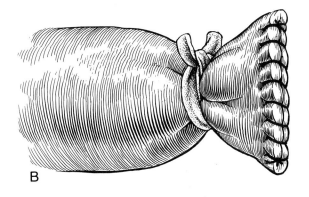

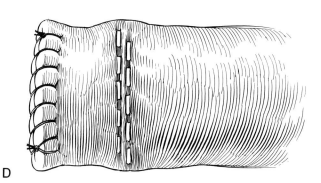

Figure 18

Methods of closing large arteries. End-on closure (*A*) and end-on closure reinforced with an umbilical tape (*B*), with an interrupted row of mattress sutures (*C*), or a row of vascular staples (*D*).

HEMOSTASIS AND ANTICOAGULATION

Having exposed and controlled the vascular segment, one is *almost* ready to enter and explore it, performing any number of disobliterative endovascular procedures through the arteriotomy (e.g., thromboembolectomy, endarterectomy, balloon dilation, and transluminal atherectomy) or to replace or bypass the involved segment using grafts and a number of anastomotic techniques. Before embarking on such definitive procedures, some method of preventing thrombosis of the temporarily occluded vessel and its immediately adjacent segments should be employed. Only the simplest, most abbreviated vascular surgical procedures can be undertaken without the need to interrupt the flow of blood temporarily. With ligation or division of major vessels, it is not ordinarily necessary to take any measures to prevent thrombus formation in the interrupted vessel. Here, it is expected that thrombus formation will eventually occur within the blind end of the vessel and propagate back as far as the origin of the last major collateral. It has been shown experimentally that, if a vessel (such as the external jugular vein of the dog) is *temporarily* occluded between two adjacent vascular loops, the blood trapped in the intervening segment will ordinarily *not* clot. However, if, in addition, this same vessel is simply opened and closed with fine silk sutures, thrombosis will commonly occur. Understandably, such segmental vascular thrombosis is even more likely in diseased vessels during the more extensive manipulations normally required in vascular surgery. In most vascular procedures the vessels are not simply opened but are explored, disobliterated, replaced, or bypassed. Therefore, to ensure restoration of flow without thromboembolic complications after an arteriotomy or a venotomy has been closed or an anastomosis has been performed, one must either prevent intravascular thrombus formation while flow is interrupted or remove all the accumulated thrombus immediately before completion of the final suture line.

If the procedure is relatively simple, accumulated thrombus may be flushed or extracted with forceps or balloon catheters just before placement or tying of the final sutures, and flow thus may be restored before further clotting recurs. Although still used as an expedient in selected circumstances, this practice carries a small but definite risk of failure—a risk that has been made largely unnecessary by the introduction of heparin anticoagulation. Except for thoracoabdominal aortic reconstructions, heparin administration during vascular cross-clamping is "routine" in most practices.

Although spontaneous clotting may be retarded by aspirin, dextran, dipyridamole, and other drugs that reduce platelet aggregation, as well as by coumarin drugs that reduce the circulating levels of clotting Factors II, VII, IX, and X, none of these drugs can be relied on to prevent intravascular thrombosis during the performance of a major vascular procedure. In comparison, in sufficient dose, heparin will render blood incoagulable at normal temperatures and pH for hours. The action of heparin is complex, affecting platelet adhesiveness, the endothelial cells' negative charge (or zeta potential), and the early phases of clotting by inhibiting the activation of Factors IX and X. However, its major action results from its union with a cofactor in the blood to form antithrombin III, which inhibits the conversion of fibrinogen to fibrin. Given intravenously, its action may persist for up to 3 to 4 hours or even longer, with higher or repeated dosage. A satisfactory level of anticoagulation for peripheral vascular procedures may be achieved within 5 minutes after the intravenous injection of 100 units per kg body weight of aqueous sodium heparin. For continued, sustained anticoagulation, as required during longer vascular procedures, half of this dose should be repeated at intervals of 1 to 1½ hours for, although some anticoagulant effect persists for two to three times this long, once one passes the half-life of heparin (about 1½ hours) some clot formation may begin, especially when dealing with diseased or damaged vessels or prosthetic surfaces. During procedures in which the blood will be exposed to large surface areas of foreign material, as during cardiopulmonary bypass, larger heparin doses (up to 300 units per kg) usually are advisable along with more precise control achieved by monitoring the activated clotting time.

Rendering the blood completely incoagulable is not without its disadvantages. Wound surfaces that would naturally remain hemostatic may bleed profusely, and spontaneous bleeding may occur elsewhere in the body; fortunately, however, these complications are extremely rare during most vascular operations. Although the greatest risk of segmental thrombosis during a vascular procedure lies in the static circulation *distal* to the point of occlusion, regional heparinization isolated to this vascular bed, by injecting the heparin downstream at the time of occlusion, cannot be practically achieved, as was once thought. Therefore, after dissection and exposure of the vessel has been carried out, including any necessary tunneling for passage of a bypass graft, and after a porous knitted Dacron graft (if it is to be used) has been preclotted, the appropriate systemic dosage of heparin (usually 100 units per kg) is injected intravenously by the anesthesiologist at the direction of the surgeon. The time is noted so that half of this dose can be repeated after 1 to 1½ hours in longer procedures.

Whenever large tissue surfaces have been exposed during the course of the dissection or extensive oozing of blood from the tissues or prosthesis occurs following completion of the anastomosis, the heparin effect may be reversed prior to wound closure by using an equivalent dose of protamine sulfate (i.e., milligram for milligram, assuming 1 mg of heparin equals 100 units), allowing for the temporal decay of the heparin given earlier. Protamine may cause hypotension (if injected too rapidly) and other adverse effects, and it may produce the opposite of the intended effect, namely hypocoagulability, if administered in a dose in excess of that needed to counteract the heparin. For this reason, the anesthesiologist usually is asked to give half of the calculated dose slowly over the first 5 minutes, then to administer additional smaller increments until the surgeon notes a decrease in oozing or the appearance of clot in the operative field. In most vascular procedures, however, protamine need not be given and, instead, the effects of administered heparin are simply allowed to wear off.

VASCULAR INCISIONS AND CLOSURES

Next to ligation or suture closure, incising and closing a vessel is the simplest of vascular techniques. It is important to be able to perform an arteriotomy or a venotomy properly, not only because of the endovascular procedures it allows but also because it can readily lead to problems if not properly performed. The major aspects for consideration are the direction of the opening and the manner of closure. Longitudinal incision is the most utilitarian. It is extensile; it allows wider inspection of the lumen; and, importantly, if the disobliterative endovascular procedure performed through it fails, it can serve as the origin for end-to-side anastomosis and bypass grafting. Its main drawback is that closure is more likely to narrow the lumen than would closure of a transverse arteriotomy. Therefore, for small arteries (less than 4 mm in diameter) in which the endovascular procedure to be performed is remote and should suffice in itself (e.g., simple embolectomy), a transverse arteriotomy is preferred. As seen in Figure 19, the initial opening

Basic Vascular Techniques

should be made with the tip of a No. 11 scalpel blade, taking care not to penetrate the back wall. Then, angled Potts scissors are employed to open the incision laterally in either direction until from 135° to 180° of the circumference has been opened, depending on the endovascular procedure contemplated. Afterward, the arteriotomy should be closed from either end toward the middle by continuous suture, except in much smaller vessels, in which interrupted sutures are employed and tied after all have been accurately placed.

As shown in Figure 20, a longitudinal arteriotomy is first opened with a sharp scalpel blade, then enlarged with angled Potts scissors, usually to at least twice the diameter of the vessel. Closure, as with all arteriotomies, is begun at each end with a double swaged-on suture placed from inside out into each corner, emerging just beyond the end of the arteriotomy and tied on the outside before using one of its ends in a running stitch carried toward the center to meet, and be tied to, the partner suture from the other end.

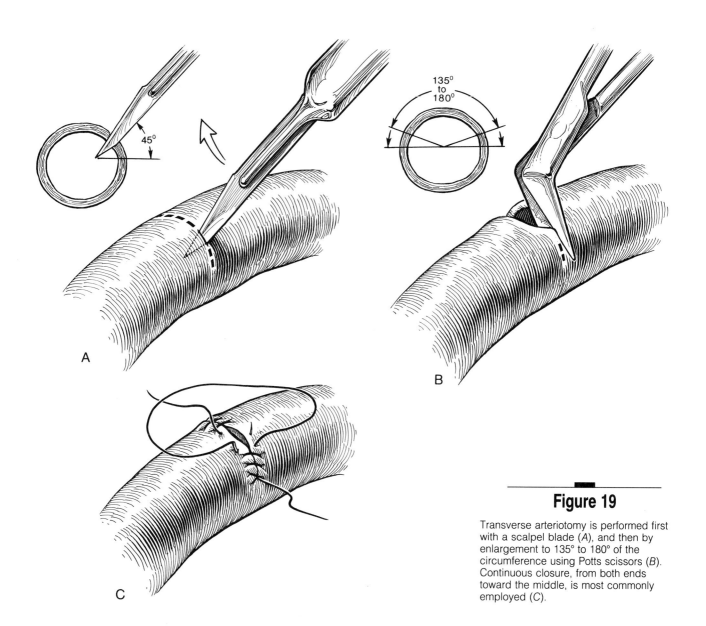

Figure 19

Transverse arteriotomy is performed first with a scalpel blade (A), and then by enlargement to 135° to 180° of the circumference using Potts scissors (B). Continuous closure, from both ends toward the middle, is most commonly employed (C).

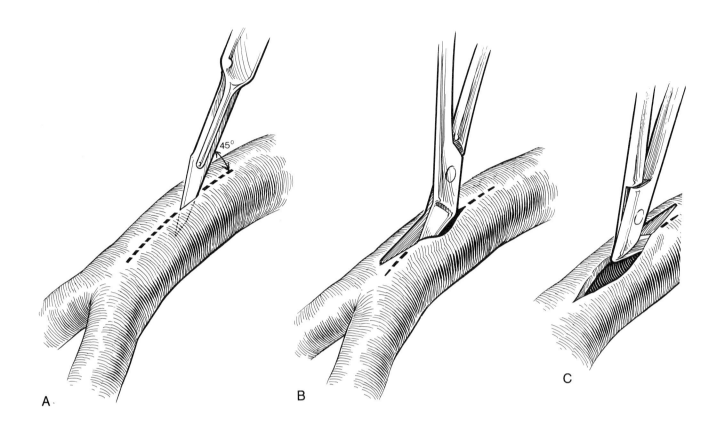

A

B

C

Figure 20

Longitudinal arteriotomy is begun with a
sharp scalpel blade and completed with
Potts scissors. Closure is performed using
continuous suture, run from each end
toward the middle.

D

E

Basic Vascular Techniques

Patch Angioplasty. Rather than closing a longitudinal arteriotomy in a smaller vessel and risking significant narrowing (as exemplified in Fig. 21*A* and *B*), patch angioplasty is preferred. Once the need is determined, the main technical considerations are the material to be used, its geometric dimensions, and the closure sequence. Autogenous tissue is best from a theoretic standpoint. If a nearby occluded artery (e.g., superficial femoral) is not available to endarterectomize and use as a patch and if a separate incision is required to harvest a superficial vein with a sufficiently thick wall to withstand arterial pressure (i.e., the upper saphenous), prosthetic material may be preferred. The use of thinner-walled veins, even the lower saphenous vein down at the ankle in some cases, has been associated with a small but definite risk of central necrosis and "blowout," resulting in catastrophic hemorrhage.

Knitted Dacron was popular as a patch 20 years ago and it is conformable, easy to sew, and, if properly preclotted, should not leak. However, it carries a greater risk of having thrombotic material adhere to its undersurface, with the buildup of a thicker, less stable pseudointima. It also has a greater infectivity potential. Therefore, the author prefers a PTFE patch as the best compromise in most cases. To achieve adequate strength, the PTFE patch should be fashioned from specially made patch material (usually 0.6 mm thickness) and not from a piece of leftover tube graft, the loose outer wrap of which can easily be disrupted and separated. Ideally, the patch should be elliptical with rounded rather than pointed ends to open up the corners of the arteriotomy. It should also be narrow enough to just compensate for the degree of narrowing that closure without a patch would cause. If it is made too wide, it will create not only a small fusiform aneurysm but also unwarranted turbulence and abnormal sheer stresses, which may lead to thromboembolic complications and aneurysm formation, respectively.

The technique is shown in Figure 22. If horizontal mattress sutures are begun at each end of the patch and carried into the corners, one end can be tied down while the other is held under traction. After the two sides of the closure have been completed from one third to halfway to the midpoint with a running suture, the other end is checked for length and trimmed to fit if necessary. Closure then begins from that end back toward the middle in similar fashion, with the continuous suture run along either side to meet and be tied to the partner suture there.

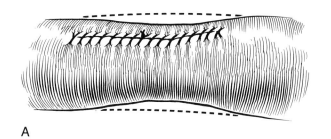

A

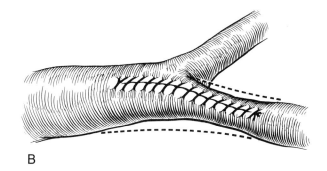

B

Figure 21

Stenosis following closure of a longitudinal arteriotomy, when it occurs in a straight arterial segment (*A*) and when carried down into a major branch (*B*).

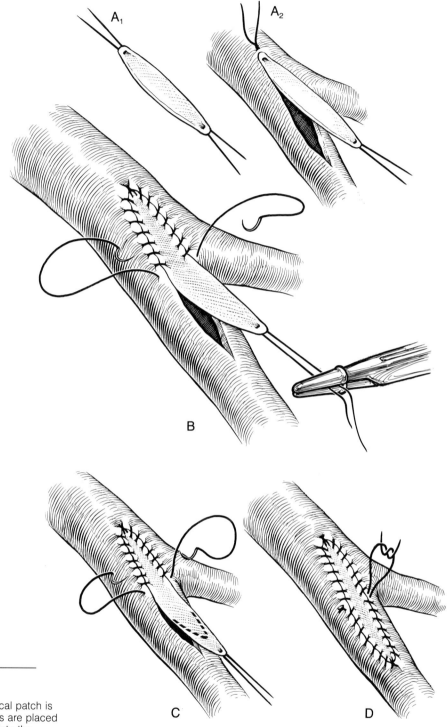

Figure 22

Patch angioplasty. A thin elliptical patch is
fashioned, and mattress sutures are placed
in both tips. One is carried on into the
corner of the arteriotomy and is tied to
begin closure, aided by traction on the other
suture. The closure is continued from each
end, along the sides of the arteriotomy, and
toward the middle, where the sutures are
tied to each other. Before beginning the
second corner the tip may need to be
trimmed for better fit.

Basic Vascular Techniques

VASCULAR ANASTOMOSES

Joining two vessels or a vessel and graft is probably the most common of all major vascular procedures. The three categorically different methods of doing this—end-to-end, end-to-side, and side-to-side anastomoses—have very different applications. Each can be modified in several ways to satisfy the particular requirements of the specific reconstructive procedure in which it is employed. The following descriptions demonstrate most of the commonly used techniques, but the experienced vascular surgeon often applies minor modifications under different circumstances or combines features of different techniques to suit the particular circumstances of the moment, rather than rigidly adhering to one of three or four standard techniques.

End-to-End Anastomosis. Conceptually, the simplest anastomosis is the perpendicular, end-to-end anastomosis shown in Figure 23. Corner sutures are placed 180° apart and, in an over-and-over fashion, are sewn toward each other. The biggest drawbacks of such an anastomosis are that (1) it requires a fair amount of mobility of the two vessel ends to allow easy and accurate placement of the sutures, especially posteriorly, and (2) it has a tendency to be constrictive if a running suture is used and drawn up tightly. Therefore, this simplest form of the technique is rarely used. It can be employed when there is adequate mobility of both ends of the vessel; for example, when one of the two "vessels" is a graft and this constitutes the first, rather than the final, anastomosis. Even then, it is the author's preference to place one suture directly posteriorly and leave the anterior suture initially untied and held loosely with a rubber-shod clamp (to avoid fraying), leaving enough slack to allow gaping of the vessel edges so that the operator can place the first two or three running stitches accurately on either side posteriorly. After that, the anterior suture may be tied and used to initiate running sutures in both directions until they have joined the "partner" at some convenient midpoint on each side. Then, rather than tying the two ends and removing the controlling clamps, this sequence is deliberately reversed. That is, the clamps are briefly and partially opened, flushing out any air or thrombus but, more importantly, allowing the continuous suture to "give" slightly and let the anastomosis expand to its full diameter before tying the two ends to each other. This maneuver is depicted in Figure 24 and is usually possible only if smooth monofilament polypropylene suture is used. Even then, the suture will slide readily only over the span of two to four "bites" in either direction. Therefore, unless helped with a fine nerve hook, this approach only suffices for intermediate-size vessels (e.g., 4 to 5 mm in diameter).

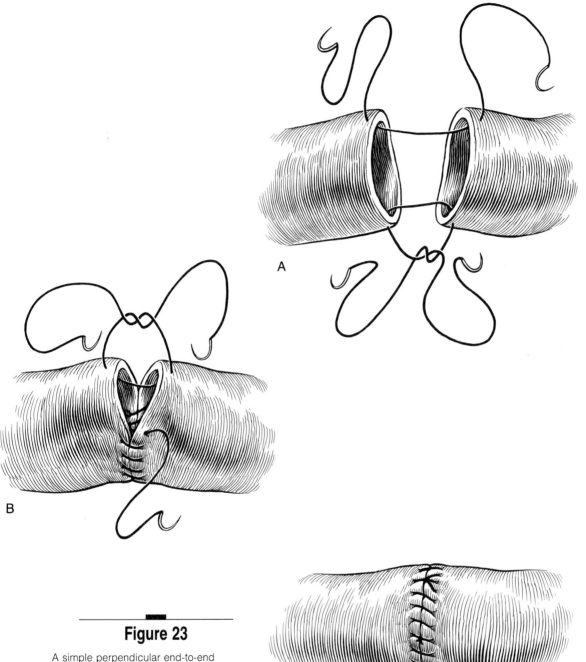

Figure 23

A simple perpendicular end-to-end anastomosis begun with two sutures 180° apart and run continuously toward each other.

Basic Vascular Techniques

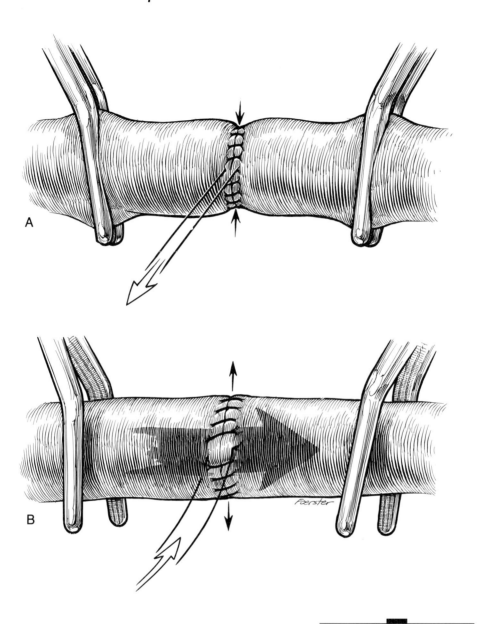

Figure 24

Pulling up and tying a continuous suture in
a perpendicular end-to-end anastomosis
may cause an anastomotic stricture (A).
Briefly releasing the clamps before tying
allows the monofilament suture to slide and
the anastomosis to expand to a fuller
diameter (B).

For larger vessels, the relatively minor degree of narrowing that continuous end-to-end anastomosis might cause is of little or no hemodynamic significance. For smaller vessels or in growing children, interrupted sutures are preferred and are often placed in horizontal mattress fashion and gently tied to allow slight eversion (Fig. 25).

When there is sufficient mobility and the vessels are of small diameter, a triangulation technique is a valuable variation to employ. As shown in Figure 26, three sutures are placed 120° apart and, using these sutures for traction and rotating the vessels, one can sew each segment of the anastomosis while it is lying directly anteriorly.

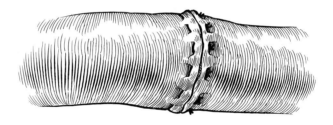

Figure 25

Interrupted vertical mattress sutures are preferred in small end-to-end perpendicular anastomoses and in growing children.

Basic Vascular Techniques

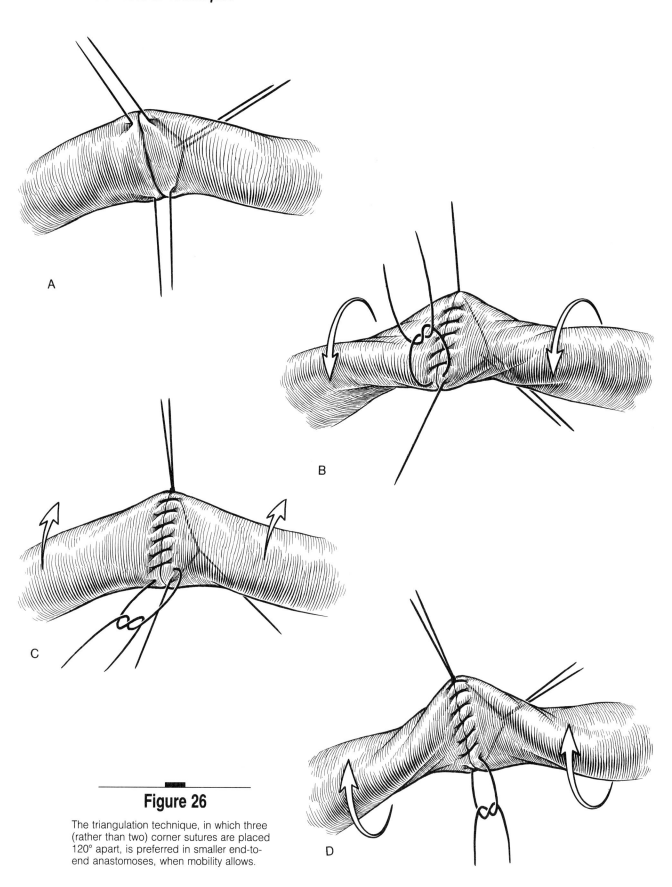

Figure 26

The triangulation technique, in which three
(rather than two) corner sutures are placed
120° apart, is preferred in smaller end-to-
end anastomoses, when mobility allows.

In general, it is best to try to avoid perpendicular end-to-end anastomoses except in the largest of vessels (e.g., the aortoiliac segment). In most cases, when there is adequate mobility of the vessel ends or one of the vessels is a graft, an oblique or bevelled anastomosis can be fashioned to minimize the risk of anastomotic narrowing (Fig. 27). As shown in Figure 28*A,* the two facing vessel ends are incised longitudinally along opposite sides (e.g., 180° apart). The angled corners created by the simple bevel cut may be removed before the anastomosis is started (Fig. 28*B*) or later (Fig. 28*E*). The two corner sutures are placed in horizontal mattress fashion and tied, and each is run in an over-and-over fashion down each side of the anastomosis toward its partner at the midpoint laterally.

Alternatively, the anastomosis can be started at one end and run circumferentially, as shown in Figure 28*C* and *D.* The latter may be preferable if mobility is more limited. However, if both corners are tied and each is run toward the other, the author prefers that the corners or "dog ears" be temporarily left untrimmed to be used to grasp the vessel edges as one places running stitches a third of the way up from either end. They are then cut to fit, removing these traumatized tips before completing the final lateral third of the anastomosis (Fig. 28*E*). This oblique end-to-end technique is particularly suited to conformable tissues (i.e., normal native vessels or vein grafts) but is not as suitable for prostheses.

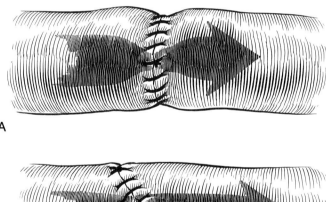

A

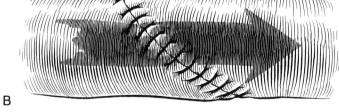

B

Figure 27

Comparison of the degree of narrowing associated with a perpendicular end-to-end technique (*A*) versus an oblique or bevelled end-to-end technique (*B*).

Basic Vascular Techniques

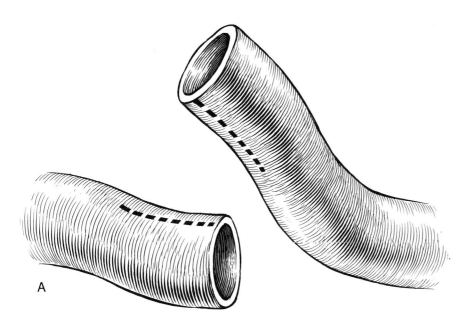

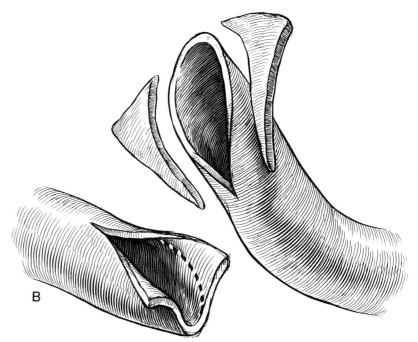

Figure 28

Technique of oblique end-to-end anastomosis. *A,* The two ends are slit 180° apart. *B,* The resultant corners and adjacent lateral edges are trimmed conservatively. *C,* Anastomosis is begun in one corner (head-to-toe) and (*D*) run to, and around, the opposite end and back toward the starting point. *E,* The other suture is run up to meet it in the middle, trimming any remaining angles to avoid "dog ears."

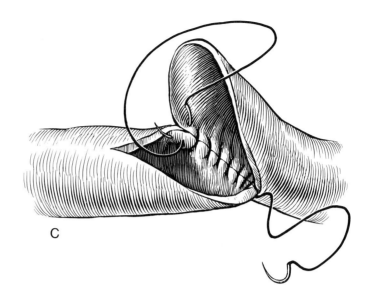

C

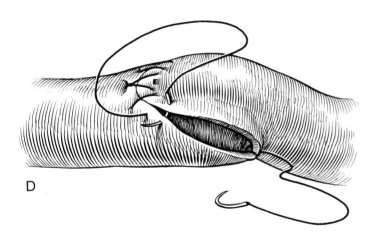

D

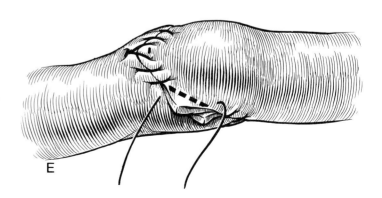

E

Basic Vascular Techniques

Because the two vessels or vessel and graft being anastomosed in this fashion are frequently of slightly different diameters, additional adjustments may need to be made. One such approach is shown in Figure 29: the larger of the two, usually the graft, is first beveled at 45°; then the smaller, usually the native vessel or vein graft, is also cut at a 45° angle, but its shorter corner is extended an additional distance, enough to accommodate the diameter difference. The angled corners are trimmed or beveled slightly to complete the matching of the circumferences of the two obliquely cut ends, before proceeding with the anastomosis in the usual manner. As long as one of the two—usually the smaller—is a reasonably pliable vessel this technique results in a satisfactory anastomosis with little angulation in the face of diameter mismatches of up to 25 to 33 percent.

An additional modification of the oblique end-to-end anastomosis is worth describing here because of its value in placing short interposition grafts in small-to-moderate sized peripheral vessels, particularly as required for trauma or small

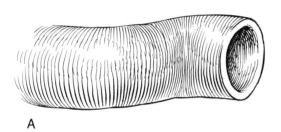 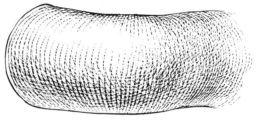

A

Figure 29

A, End-to-end anastomosis between a smaller artery (left) and a larger prosthesis (right). Both are beveled 45° (*B*). The smaller conduit is slit longitudinally, enough to accommodate the diameter mismatch. *C*, The anastomosis is performed with continuous suture beginning from each end and running toward the other. *D*, The completed anastomosis shows no significant angulation or narrowing.

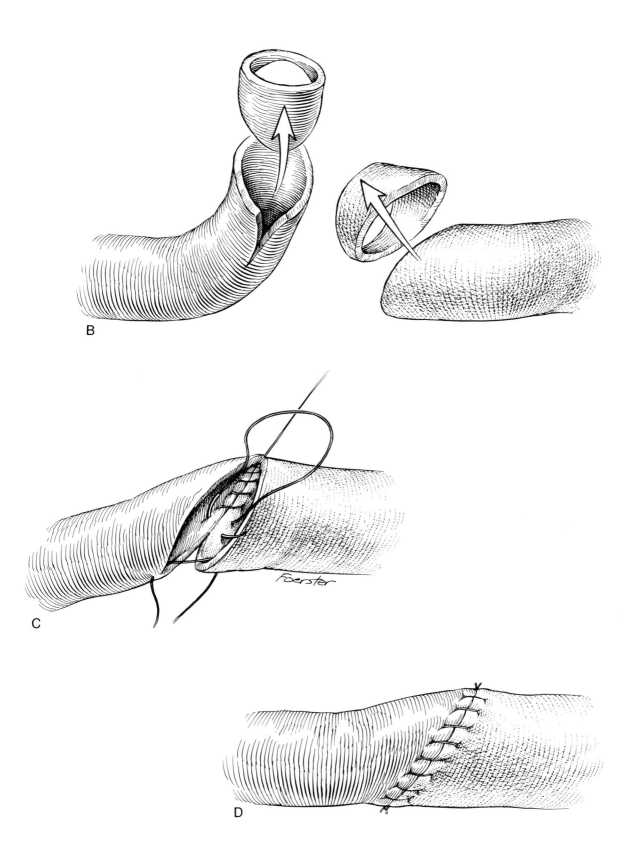

B

C

Foerster

D

Basic Vascular Techniques

aneurysm (Fig. 30*A* and *B*). If one simply transects the vessel at each end above and below the injured or diseased segment, the vessel ends will retract and the correct distance between them is forever lost (Fig. 30*C*). Even if this distance is accurately measured beforehand, the need to pull the vessel ends together accurately and steadily enough to allow the anastomosis to be performed without tension requires an assistant to retract inward with vascular clamps on each vessel end. This not only may be traumatic, but also completely occupies one assistant. As shown in Figure 30*D*, the author's preferred technique in this situation is to leave a strip of the posterior wall of the injured or diseased vessel approximately 10 to 20 percent of the circumference, which will exactly preserve the intervening length without the need for inward traction by vascular clamps. The two vessel ends are beveled outward at 45°, allowing oblique anastomoses. Each anastomosis

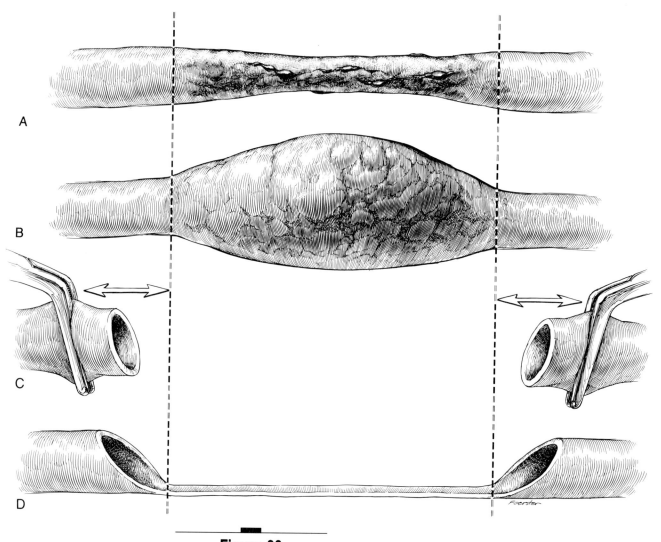

Figure 30

A and B, Dotted lines show segments of injured artery and aneurysm, respectively, to be replaced with an interposition graft. *C,* The effect of segmental resection—namely, retraction of adjacent vessel ends and loss of proper length without traction on vascular clamps. *D,* Leaving a strip of arterial wall intact preserves proper length and makes traction on clamps unnecessary.

is begun with a horizontal mattress suture placed from the outside in, beginning at the corner adjacent to the posterior strip and continuing into the inside of the graft (Fig. 30E). After this suture is tied, it is run along each side of the anastomosis to some convenient meeting point with the other side before completion (Fig. 30F). If, in spite of these precautions, the interposition graft is still a little too long when completed (Fig. 30G), the posterior strip can simply be cut at one or both ends, having served its purpose, allowing the natural elasticity of the adjacent artery to recoil enough to make a final length correction and achieve a straight configuration (Fig. 30H).

Figure 30 *Continued*

E and F, Anastomotic technique is demonstrated. *G,* To achieve proper tension, the posterior strip is later divided, straightening out the anastomosis, as shown in *H.*

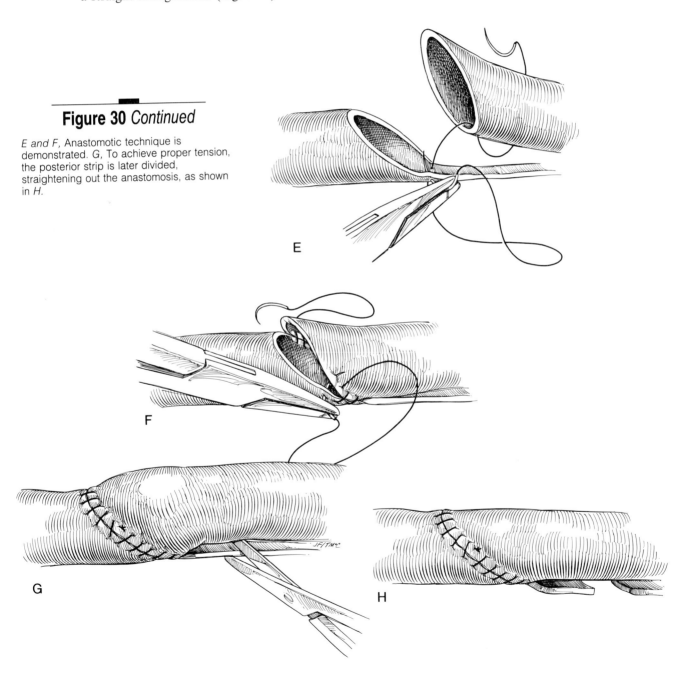

Basic Vascular Techniques

As commonly performed in the repair of larger (e.g., aortic) aneurysms, an end-to-end anastomosis may be performed to the rim or "neck" of the aneurysm—that is, the junction between normal artery and aneurysm, *from the inside* (Fig. 31A through *E*). It is probably the most common clinical application of a perpendicular end-to-end anastomosis, and the introduction and popularization of this intraluminal approach by Creech and by DeBakey revolutionized aortic aneurysm surgery. After opening the aneurysm longitudinally and "T-ing" the ends, as shown in Figure 31A, mural thrombus is removed and (lumbar) collaterals are suture ligated. Then, a continuous suture, deeply placed to incorporate a double thickness of arterial wall, is begun in the posterior midline *(B)* and run around either side, up onto the anterior aspect toward the center *(C, D, and E)*. A similar technique is used for the distal anastomosis.

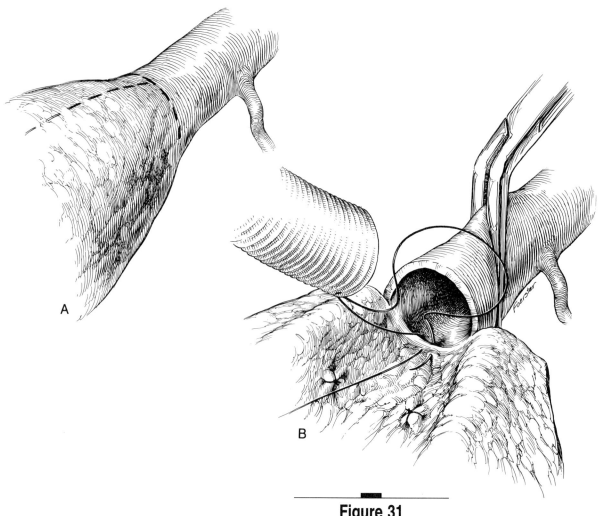

Figure 31

Classic intraluminal aneurysm repair is shown with (*A*) the arteriotomy line, (*B*) the posterior midline mattress suture to begin with, and (*C, D, and E*) the circumferential running suture around both sides to meet at the midline anteriorly.

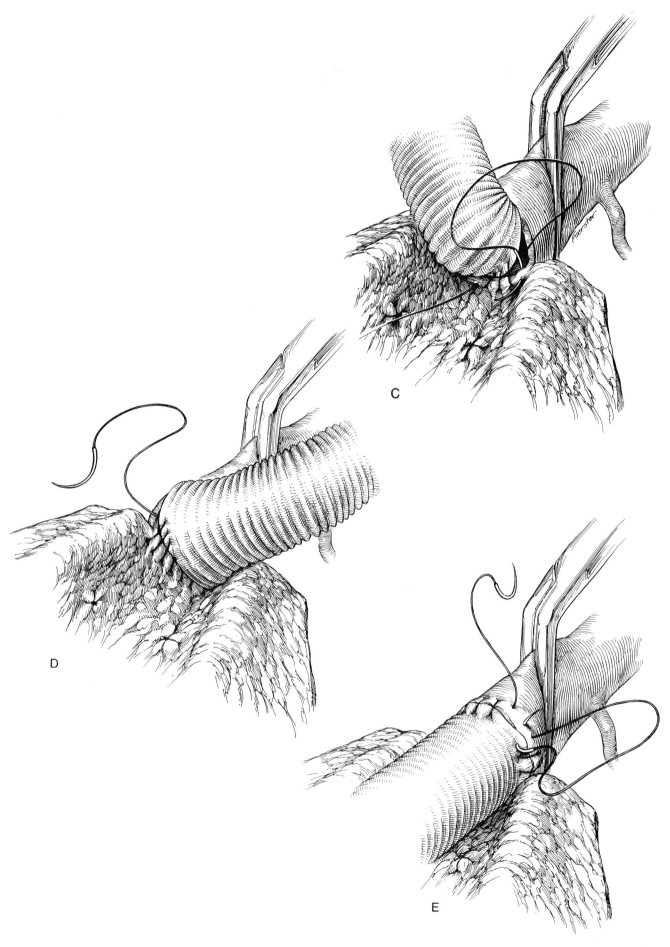

C

D

E

Basic Vascular Techniques

End-to-Side Anastomosis. The end-to-side anastomosis is the most common prototype employed in arterial reconstructive surgery and is the basis for most bypass grafting which, in principle, attempts to provide a normal-caliber conduit for blood to flow around the diseased segment without having to dissect out and remove the latter and without interrupting any residual flow traversing that segment or the collaterals emanating from it. End-to-side anastomosis is mainly used in occlusive rather than aneurysmal disease. If used in the latter circumstance, the aneurysmal segment must be excluded from arterial inflow by appropriate ligature or other obliterative techniques. This bypass technique presents the further advantages of allowing one to work with normal or, at least, less diseased vessels above and below the lesion and of approaching them at convenient, accessible, and familiar sites of exposure. By using the end-to-side anastomotic configuration, even remote bypass still preserves pulsatile flow into each end of the bypassed segment. In comparison with bypasses with end-to-end anastomoses, one is no worse off hemodynamically if the bypass occludes and is better off if it becomes infected, in that graft removal and suture line closure (usually with autogenous patch angioplasty) usually restores flow to preoperative levels.

The relative dimensions of the end-to-side anastomosis deserve some comment. Theoretically, the more acutely angled and longer the anastomosis, the better, but from a practical standpoint an opening twice the diameter of the native vessel or graft and a 30° angle of anastomosis are close to ideal (Fig. 32A). In certain circumstances (e.g., the proximal anastomosis of an axillofemoral bypass or a radiocephalic arteriovenous fistula), a less acute angle, up to 75°, is acceptable (Fig. 32B).

Depending on its diameter, the end of one vessel or, most commonly, the graft, is either beveled at 30° (for larger vessels) or slit along one side with the corners trimmed (for smaller vessels). For vessels of intermediate size, a combination of a 45° bevel and a short slit may be used to prepare it for anastomosis (Fig. 33A and B). A longitudinal arteriotomy is then made in the side of the recipient vessel to match this opening in longitudinal dimension. The anastomosis is begun with a horizontal mattress at the upper end of the cut end, or "heel" (Fig. 33C), and continued along each side about a third of the way toward the middle. Then another mattress suture secures the tip, or "toe," of the graft into the other corner of the recipient vessel (Fig. 33D), and the anastomosis is completed with a running suture back along each side to meet and be tied to its partner, trimming the excess cornered edges to fit (Fig. 33E). When a vein graft of smaller diameter than the recipient artery has been slit and trimmed in the described fashion (Fig. 34A), the completed, stretched-out anastomosis takes on the characteristic "cobra-head" configuration for which it is named (Fig. 34B and C).

The suturing sequence here is similar to that already described for oblique end-to-end anastomoses. As diagrammed in Figure 35, it consists of starting first with the lower (underneath) corner (or heel) and continuing along each side one third to one half of the way before beginning with another double swaged-on suture at the superior corner (or toe) and sewing back along each edge to join the other (partner) suture somewhere at the midlateral point (Fig. 35A). Though the popular practice of stopping on one side at the midlateral point and then running the other suture three quarters of the circumference around the toe to meet it (Fig. 35B) is perfectly acceptable in some settings, doing the anastomosis in "quarters," starting from each end, is the safest and most accurate technique, as it takes advantage of the ease of doing the most difficult aspects first. Starting at the opposite end, or toe, would make the heel difficult if not impossible to complete. It might be likened to painting (sewing) oneself into a corner. Even

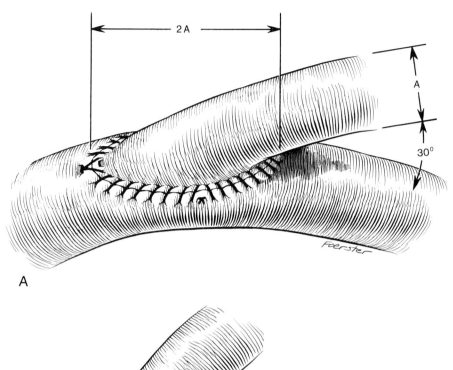

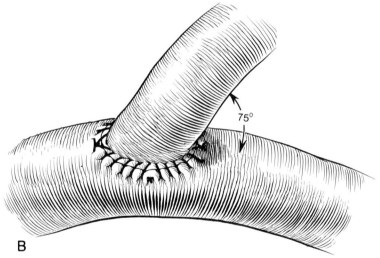

A

B

Figure 32

A, Ideal dimensions of an end-to-side anastomosis, an acute (about 30°) angle of entry and a 2:1 ratio of anastomosis to graft diameter. *B,* A greater angle, up to 75°, is acceptable when dictated by anatomic considerations.

Basic Vascular Techniques

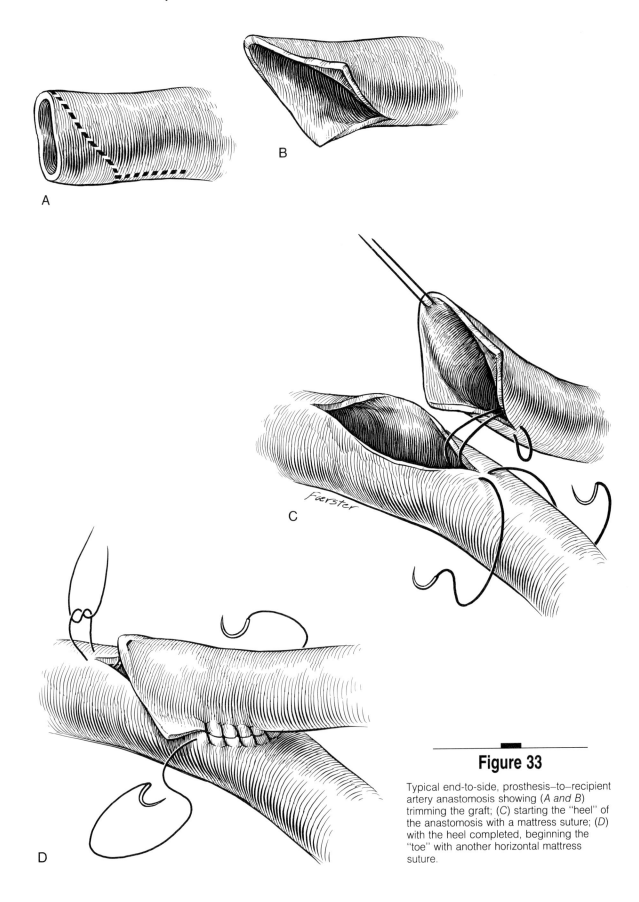

Figure 33

Typical end-to-side, prosthesis–to–recipient artery anastomosis showing (*A and B*) trimming the graft; (*C*) starting the "heel" of the anastomosis with a mattress suture; (*D*) with the heel completed, beginning the "toe" with another horizontal mattress suture.

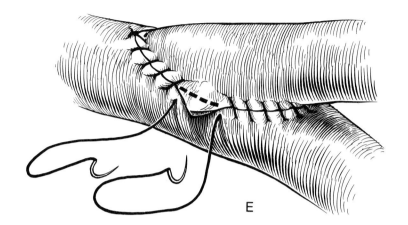

Figure 33 *Continued*

(*E*) excess edges to be trimmed before completion.

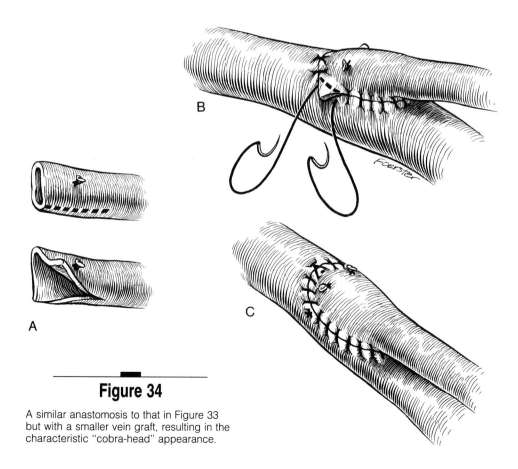

Figure 34

A similar anastomosis to that in Figure 33 but with a smaller vein graft, resulting in the characteristic "cobra-head" appearance.

Basic Vascular Techniques

tying the toe down at the same time as the heel can make suturing at the latter end unnecessarily difficult. By waiting to tie down the toe *after* the sutures from the heel have progressed well along each side, one has the opportunity to make adjustments for proper fitting of that end of the anastomosis, either trimming the tip of the graft or extending the arteriotomy, as shown in Figure 36*A* and *B*. It also allows the final few sutures to be safely placed blindly (i.e., without seeing both the inner and outer aspects of each vessel), laterally where there is the least chance and consequence of error. In contrast, improper depth or spacing at the

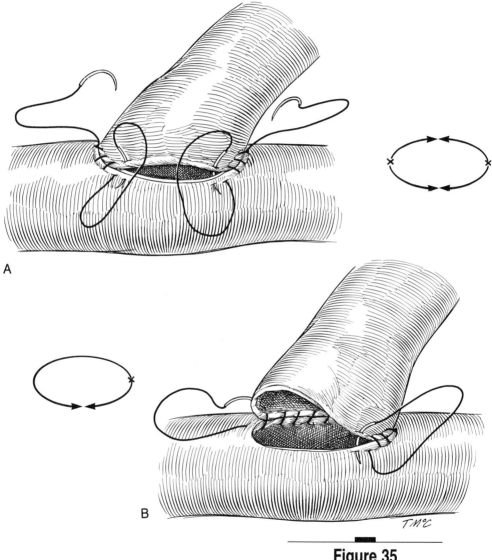

A

B

T.M°C.

Figure 35

Optional suture sequences for end-to-side anastomoses. *A,* The two ends are run toward each other along each side, heel first and toe last. Performing the anastomosis in quarters, in this fashion, is safer and more accurate. *B,* Doing one quarter, then three quarters, starting from the heel with a single double-needled suture, is popular and perfectly acceptable when exposure is excellent.

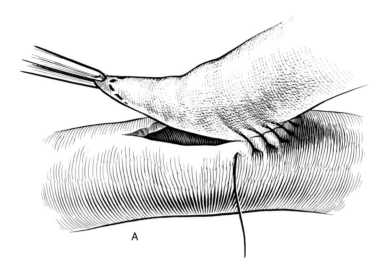

A

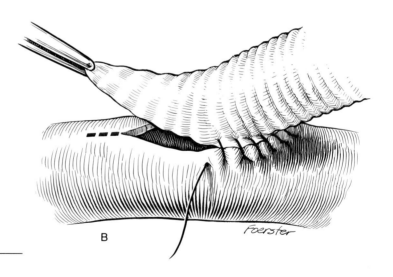

B

Foerster

Figure 36

The advantages of the heel-first, toe-last
sequence are illustrated. A final length
adjustment is allowed either by trimming the
tip (toe) *(A)* or by extending the arteriotomy
(B).

Basic Vascular Techniques

toe or heel can lead to narrowing at the most critical outflow point of the anastomosis or inaccessible anastomotic bleeding, respectively.

Technical Tips: By using vertical mattress sutures at each corner to begin with (à la Kunlin), and by penetrating each edge *perpendicularly with equal depth bites* as one progresses away from each corner, the lateral edges are encouraged to evert, thereby allowing accurate, even, through-and-through needle passages to be made blindly along the lateral aspects of the anastomosis (Fig. 37). Spacing and depth of suture placement will vary on either side of the traditional advice of "1 mm apart, 1 mm deep," depending on the size and thickness of the vessels, but even spacing and equal depth from *each* edge will minimize suture line leakage through uneven gaps or overbiting edges. *Perpendicular* needle penetration to the edge of the vessel or graft not only encourages eversion but also allows easier penetration of plaques and Dacron knit or weave and makes smaller holes in PTFE grafts. Pushing the needle through evenly and steadily, and following the curve of the needle rather than torquing or levering it as commonly taught with skin, fascial, or gastrointestinal closures, will obviate much of the needle hole bleeding seen with PTFE grafts and friable arteriosclerotic vessels. The needle should always penetrate the arteriosclerotic vessel from the inside out, to avoid pushing adjacent plaques inward and creating intimal flaps (Fig. 38). Thus, the traditional advice of "outside-in on the graft, inside-out on the artery" is sound. This will require a backhand penetration on the needle in the side of the anastomosis away from the surgeon. This may be a little awkward at first for beginners, but with experience, vascular surgeons, like good tennis players, soon execute backhand and forehand with comparable skill.

Prosthetic grafts are not usually beveled in the same manner as a vein graft or native vessel. The Gore-Tex PTFE graft has a thin outer helical wrap, which gives it necessary extra strength but which may also lift off or fray when cut with scissors. Therefore, it is better held with a slightly curved hemostat or clamp (tonsil or Crile) and cut along the inner edge of the curve of the clamp with a scalpel blade (Fig. 39A). Dacron may be shaped with scissors in a number of ways. It may be simply cut across at an appropriate angle—usually between 30° and 50°—with the tip slightly trimmed or rounded off. If an anastomosis close to 45° is desired, a lazy-S configuration, shown as "a" in Figure 39B, may also be used to give sufficient length. If a flatter anastomosis is wanted—one with an angle closer to 30°—a gentle French curve may be used, starting at 60° at the tip and continuing to slope upward, becoming more acutely angled toward the base (i.e., 30° or less). This variation is shown as "b" in Figure 39B, with the resulting anastomoses shown in "a" and "b" in Figure 39C.

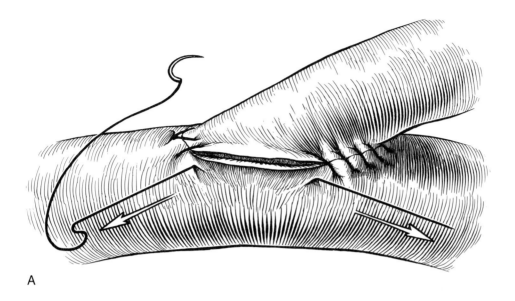

A

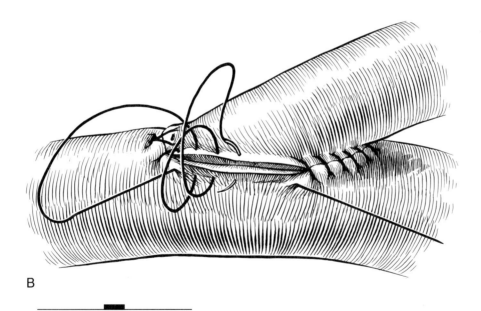

B

Figure 37

Even, perpendicular "bites" progressing away from the heel and toe (A) and traction encourage eversion (B), which allows the lateral sutures to be rapidly and blindly placed with accuracy.

Basic Vascular Techniques

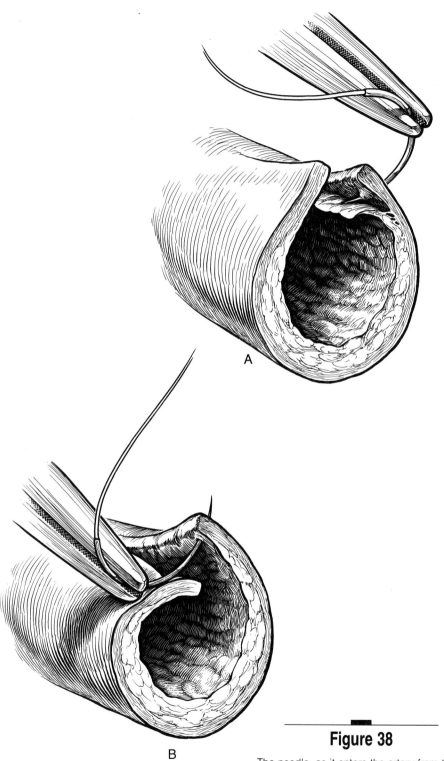

A

B

Figure 38

The needle, as it enters the artery from the outside inward, may push the edge of a plaque in, creating an internal flap or dissection, or both, as shown in *A*. The advice, "always inside out on the artery," as shown in *B*, is intended to avoid this problem.

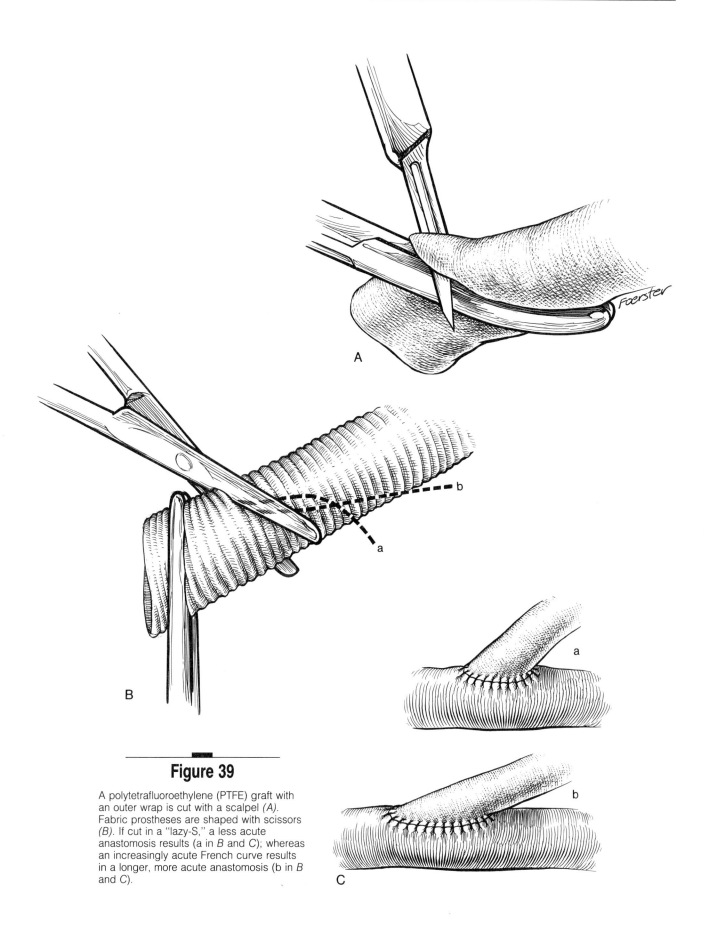

Figure 39

A polytetrafluoroethylene (PTFE) graft with
an outer wrap is cut with a scalpel (A).
Fabric prostheses are shaped with scissors
(B). If cut in a "lazy-S," a less acute
anastomosis results (a in B and C); whereas
an increasingly acute French curve results
in a longer, more acute anastomosis (b in B
and C).

Basic Vascular Techniques

Rounding or squaring off the tip of the graft is a common maneuver used to open up or widen the distal corner of the anastomosis, much as one tries to achieve with patch angioplasty (see Fig. 22). Another technique to avoid narrowing at the insertion of the tip of graft involves squaring off the graft tip and T-ing the end of the arteriotomy with a short transverse incision. This technique is shown in Figure 40, where Teflon pledgets are also shown buttressing the tip of the anastomosis. The latter is not often necessary. In fact, it is only occasionally used by the author when there is concern about tension between the graft and the native vessel at its tip. When the arterial wall seems unduly friable, as in dealing with aneurysmal degeneration, one to three pledget-reinforced interrupted mattress sutures may be placed across the tip or toe of the graft and then a continuous suture employed to complete the rest of the lateral edge of the anastomosis.

The use of interrupted sutures, with the exception of two or three sutures across the tip to ensure accurate placement in smaller anastomoses, is relatively uncommon with end-to-side anastomosis, as compared with end-to-end anastomosis. However, when exposure is limited (such as a popliteal anastomosis at knee level approached through an above-knee incision and bending the knees to preserve muscle and tendon attachments), accurate placement of sutures may be quite difficult. Here, the technique of first placing several continuous sutures at the heel before drawing them tightly into place, and then repeating this at the toe of the anastomosis, has considerable merit. It is called "parachuting" by some, presumably because, like a parachute, the graft is tethered by multiple parallel strands of suture (shrouds), as it descends to its final resting place. It is important not to tangle these strands. In this technique, shown in Figure 41, one begins with a horizontal mattress suture, then makes two additional over-and-over graft-to-vessel needle passages on either side, using a nerve hook or small right-angle clamp to keep the shrouds from tangling or crossing and to maintain even tension and length. Then, by pulling up on each end of the slick monofilament polypropylene suture, the graft is drawn down into place, utilizing the nerve hook to assist in the orderly drawing down of each loop of the suture.

Occasionally, an end-to-side anastomosis will need to be performed with a much less acute angle of entry because of limited mobility of one or both vessels, for example, in the end-of-vein to side-of-artery anastomoses in creating angioaccess arteriovenous fistulas. Commonly, the posterior suture line in these anastomoses is difficult to place from the outside of the lumen. Figure 42 shows one approach the author uses in this situation. The two corner sutures are first placed, but only the one at the most acutely angled end is tied down—on the outside as usual. Then, one of the suture ends is selected and the needle is passed from the *outside in* into the corner on the *upper edge* of the *posterior* suture line (Fig. 42A). With the suture now on the inside and the corner tightened, the posterior suture line is performed in continuous over-and-over fashion, running toward the other corner. The amount of slack at this corner is controlled to allow it to be approached by the suture from the other end and securely closed with accurate suture placement. At this point, the traction suture at the opposite end can be tied down to itself (Fig. 42B) and then tied to the other suture (Fig. 42C) or the traction suture can be simply continued around the corner onto the anterior suture line to reach the midpoint before the other end of the original suture is used to complete the final quadrant of the anastomosis, finishing in the midline anteriorly (Fig. 42D and E).

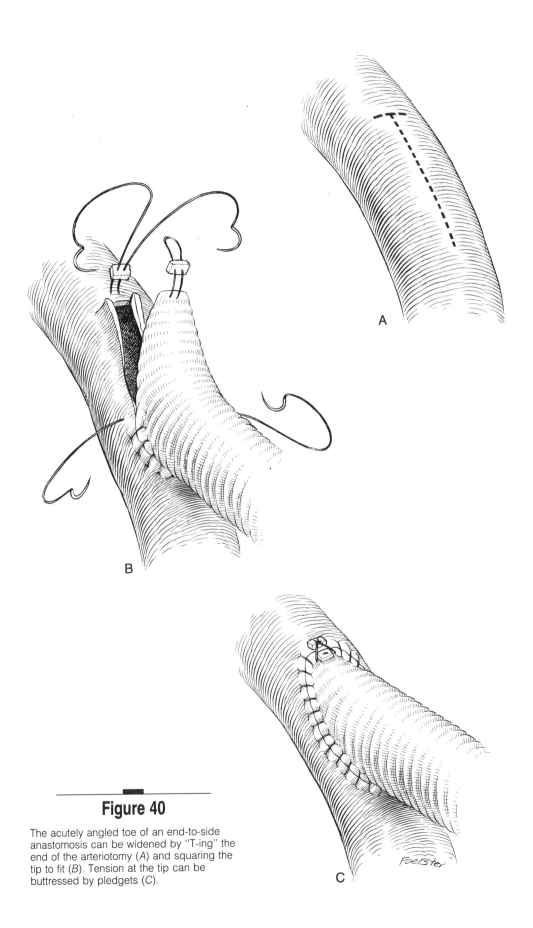

Figure 40

The acutely angled toe of an end-to-side anastomosis can be widened by "T-ing" the end of the arteriotomy (A) and squaring the tip to fit (B). Tension at the tip can be buttressed by pledgets (C).

Basic Vascular Techniques

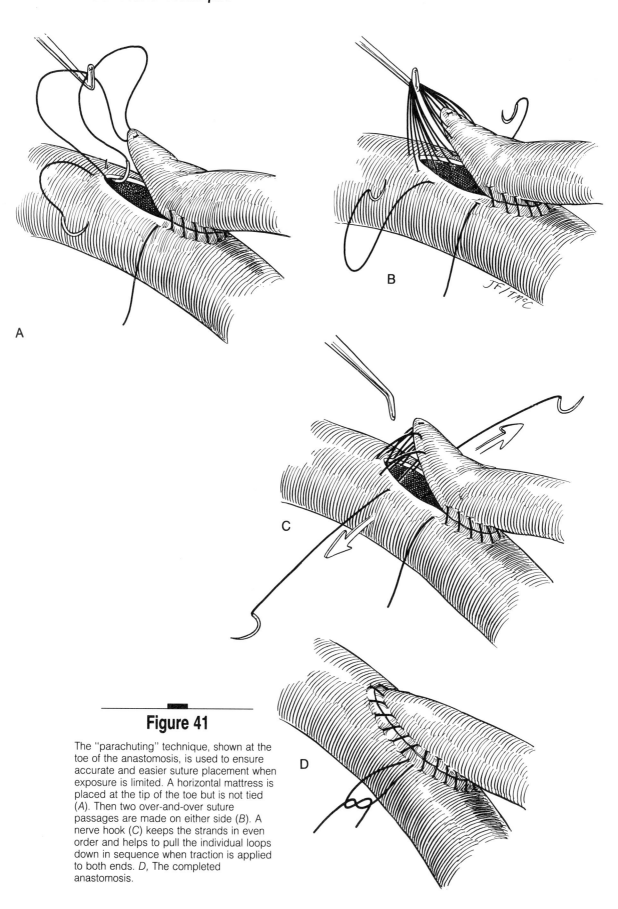

A

B

C

Figure 41

The "parachuting" technique, shown at the toe of the anastomosis, is used to ensure accurate and easier suture placement when exposure is limited. A horizontal mattress is placed at the tip of the toe but is not tied (A). Then two over-and-over suture passages are made on either side (B). A nerve hook (C) keeps the strands in even order and helps to pull the individual loops down in sequence when traction is applied to both ends. D, The completed anastomosis.

D

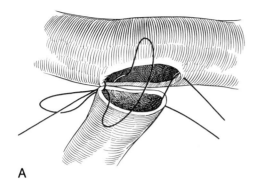

A

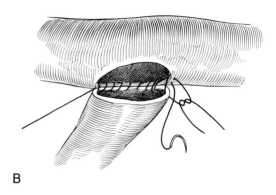

B

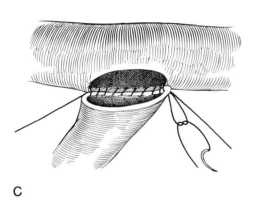

C

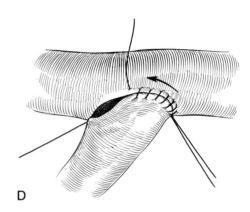

D

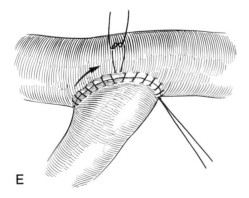

E

Figure 42

An end-to-side technique used when there is limited mobility of the vessel or graft end. *A,* Sutures are placed at each corner, but only one is tied down. *B,* It is then used to sew the posterior suture line from the inside. Leaving the other suture untied but under moderate tension allows the second corner to be rounded with accurate suture placement. *C,* After the second suture is tied, the anterior aspect of the anastomosis is completed from either end toward the middle (*D, E*), as described in the text.

Basic Vascular Techniques

Another approach that is useful in end-to-side anastomoses when the angle of entry is closer to perpendicular than usual and there is limited access to the far side of the anastomosis (typified by subclavian or vertebral to carotid bypass or transposition anastomoses) is shown in Figure 43. The suture line is begun in the middle of the posterior aspect and simply run around either edge to the corner before completion of the anterior aspect of the anastomosis in the usual fashion. This is not a difficult technique if one is dealing with pliable, conformable vessels, particularly if one cuts a circular or an elliptical opening in the recipient vessel (sometimes conveniently created with an aortic punch). The key to success is gauging the correct size of the opening and stretching out the donor vessel to conform evenly to its circumference, as one applies the continuous suture.

"Island Inclusion" Technique: One other important variation of the end-to-side anastomosis is also performed from the inside. This special technique involves the suturing of an elliptical island or button containing the orifices of one or more visceral arteries into the side of a Dacron graft, usually being placed for reconstruction of an aortic aneurysm. This approach is preferred to sewing the divided end of the artery directly onto the graft because of several advantages: (1) it requires less dissection of the branch vessel; (2) it allows a bigger anastomosis; (3) the anastomosis is stronger; and (4) it provides the opportunity to incorporate multiple adjacent orifices in one anastomosis. In thoracoabdominal reconstruction at least, it also saves precious time.

One common variation in this technique, employed to include multiple branch orifices, is shown in Figure 44. After fashioning an elliptical opening of appropriate size in the graft, designed to fit an imaginary island reaching about 3 mm beyond each of the orifices (Fig. 44*A*), a continuous suture is begun at the upper end, just above the most proximal visceral artery orifice. Then, using large hemostatic bites penetrating through and through a double thickness of aortic wall for added strength (Fig. 44*B*), a continuous suture is continued down around the lower edge of these orifices and then, switching to the outside, started up along the anterior suture line in front of each orifice there. Once the corner is turned, the other end of the suture is started down the anterior suture line to meet its partner (Fig. 44*C*). This is particularly suited to incorporation of the celiac axis and superior mesenteric and right renal arteries into one anastomosis. As popularized by Stanley Crawford, this revolutionized thoracoabdominal aneurysm repair.

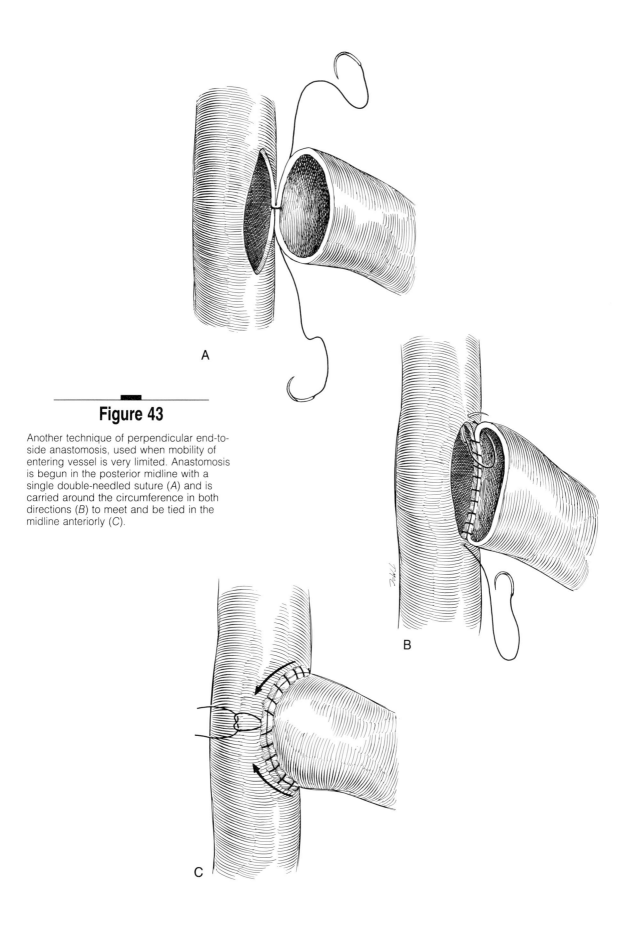

Figure 43

Another technique of perpendicular end-to-side anastomosis, used when mobility of entering vessel is very limited. Anastomosis is begun in the posterior midline with a single double-needled suture (A) and is carried around the circumference in both directions (B) to meet and be tied in the midline anteriorly (C).

Basic Vascular Techniques

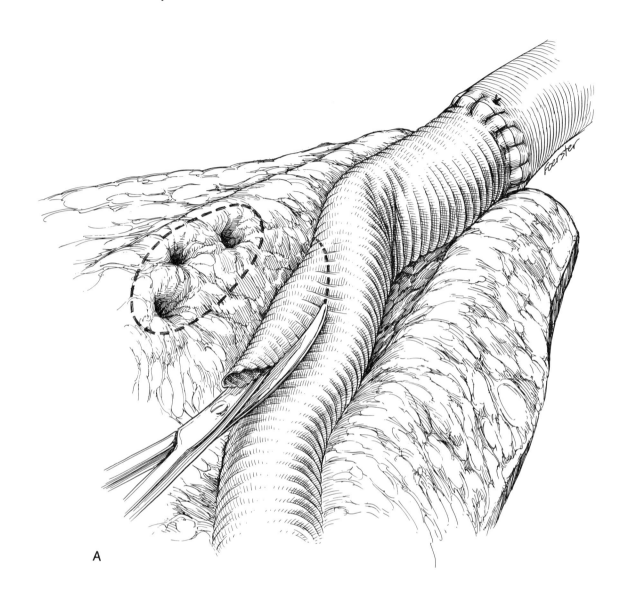

A

Figure 44

Classic end-to-side anastomosis of an aortic
orifice "island" into the side of an aortic
Dacron graft, showing fashioning the
elliptical opening to fit the imaginary island
(A), performing the back row *(B)*, and, after
rounding the lower end of the island,
completing the final quarter of the
anastomosis with the other end of the
suture, anteriorly *(C)*.

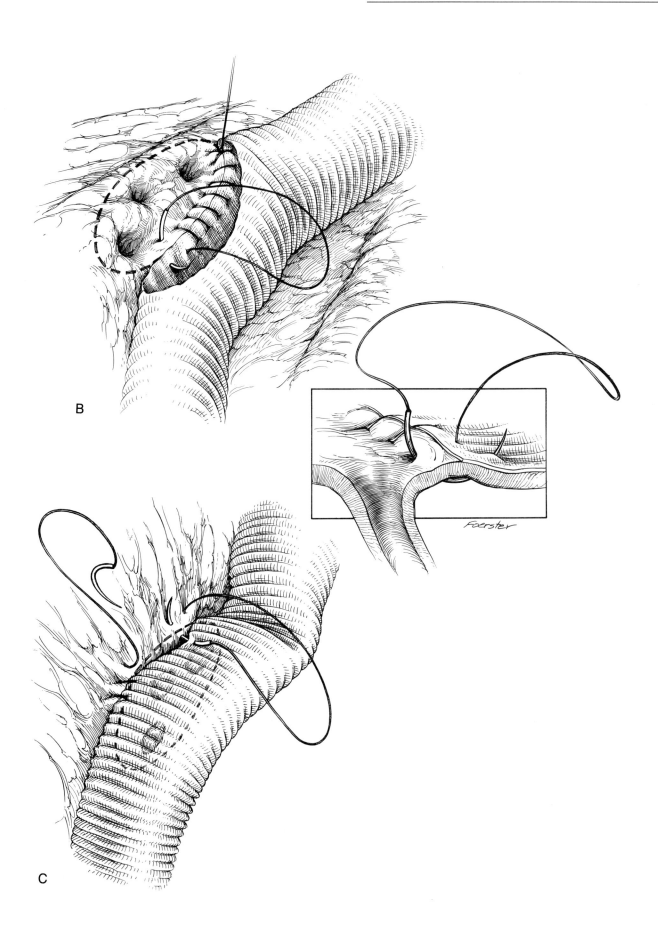

Basic Vascular Techniques

Alternatively, as shown in Figure 45, a button of aortic wall surrounding a single branch orifice can be cut out, almost like a Carrel patch, and sutured circumferentially into an appropriately sized opening in the graft. This technique, commonly used to reanastomose the inferior mesenteric artery to a Dacron graft during aortic aneurysm repair, allows a wider anastomotic orifice than direct suture of the native vessel. This anastomotic button can be sewn more precisely and can be brought *to* the graft rather than the reverse. Occasionally endarterectomy to remove occlusive disease at the orifice of such major branches may be necessary before anastomosis.

Side-to-Side Anastomosis. The side-to-side anastomosis is no longer commonly performed in clinical vascular surgery. The best known examples of this technique probably are the side-to-side portacaval shunt, the Potts and Waterston aortopulmonary anastomoses, and the arteriovenous fistulas for angioaccess. Occasionally, favorable anatomy and exposure will allow this technique to be applied to left subclavian-carotid anastomosis, very low in the neck (almost in the thoracic outlet). Finally, it may be used in some circumstances as the middle anastomosis in a sequential bypass of multilevel occlusive disease employing a single graft.

In most such instances, one can employ most of the variations in technique described for end-to-side anastomosis. A special exception is the side-to-side shunt performed between two large pliable vessels without interrupting flow in either (e.g., portacaval shunt). For this anastomosis, a curved, spoon-shaped, or angled Satinsky vascular clamp may be placed laterally on adjacent segments of the two vessels to be anastomosed, aided by traction on stay sutures (Fig. 46A). Then, after matching longitudinal incisions are made in each segment (Fig. 46B), the adjacent openings can be sutured together with continuous suture, the posterior suture line being performed intraluminally (Fig. 46C). If problems are encountered because the posterior or inner suture line gets in the way while the anterior or outer suture line is being performed, the posterior suture line can be made to drop away from the anterior suture line by holding up the two sutures and briefly releasing the Satinsky clamp (Fig. 46D and E).

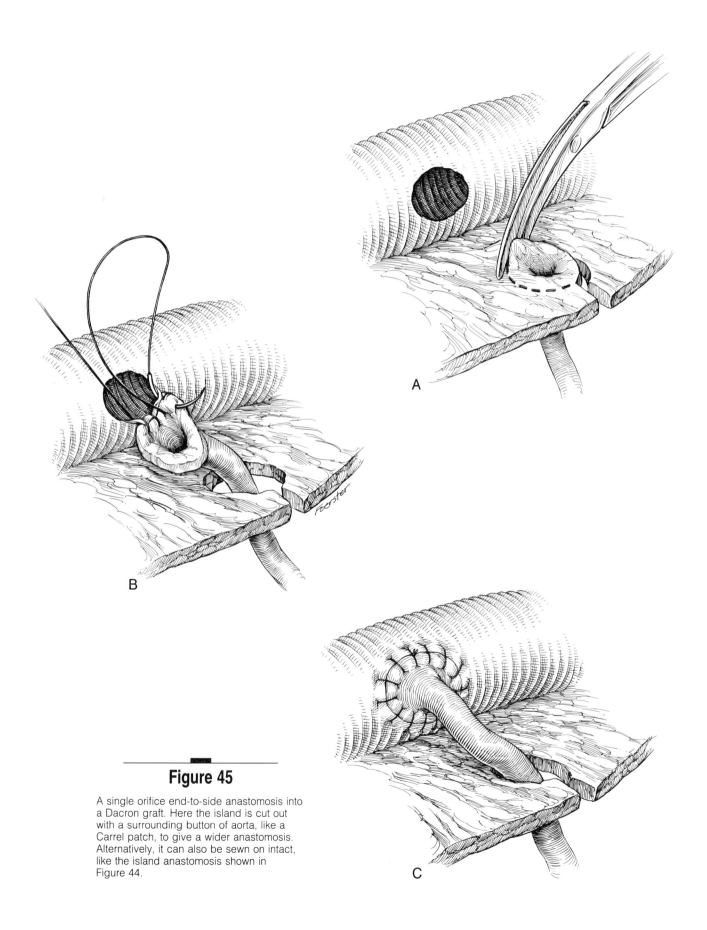

A

B

C

Figure 45

A single orifice end-to-side anastomosis into a Dacron graft. Here the island is cut out with a surrounding button of aorta, like a Carrel patch, to give a wider anastomosis. Alternatively, it can also be sewn on intact, like the island anastomosis shown in Figure 44.

Basic Vascular Techniques

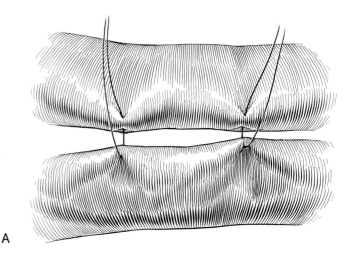

A

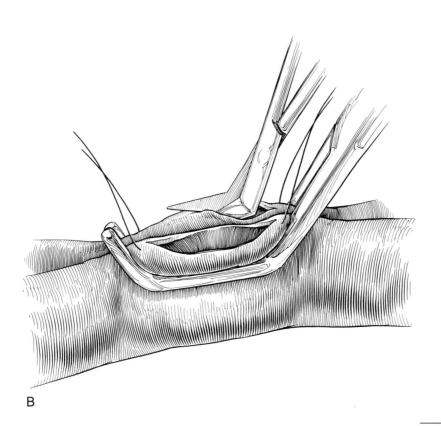

B

Figure 46

A technique of side-to-side anastomosis
between two large (e.g., portal and caval)
veins in which a single partially occluding
vascular clamp is applied to both vessels
simultaneously with the aid of stay sutures.
Briefly releasing the clamp after beginning
each end of the anterior suture line will allow
the posterior suture line to drop down out of
the way to facilitate completion of the
anastomosis.

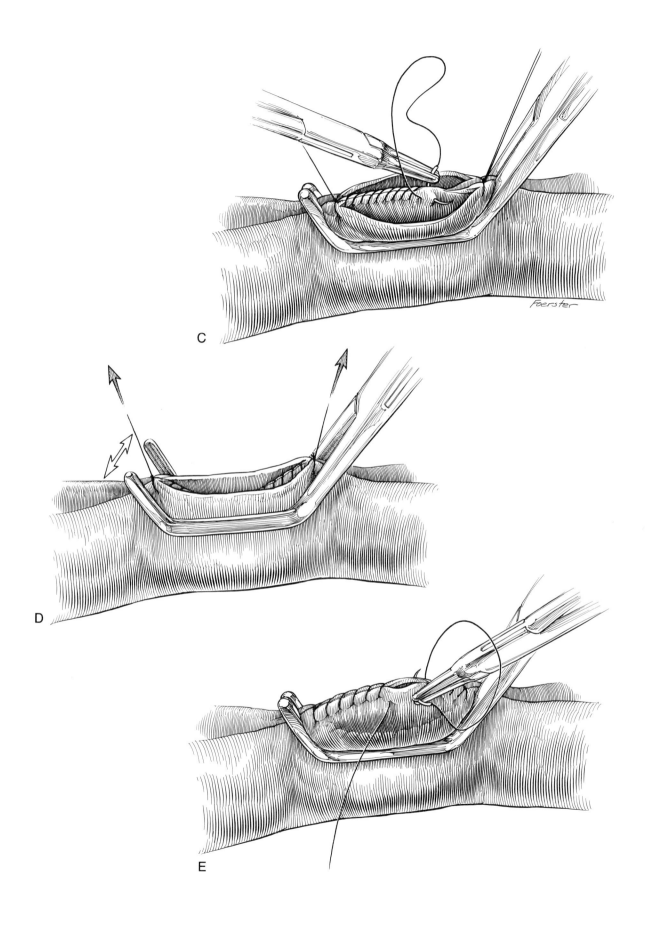

C

D

E

Basic Vascular Techniques

The practice of sewing the posterior or "away" half of the anastomosis intraluminally often is dictated by limited exposure and lack of mobility of the vessels being joined. In venous anastomosis, it is particularly advantageous to evert the suture line to allow as little suture material as possible to be exposed to the lumen of the vessel. Ideally, running horizontal mattress suture should be used here, but this is almost impossible to place from below. Starzl has described an innovative method by which this can be performed intraluminally. This is depicted in Figure 47 (see page 72) and usually requires the application of two parallel vascular clamps, rather than one clamp on both vessels, to provide extra mobility. After the corner sutures are placed (Fig. 47*A*), one of the needled ends of the suture is introduced into the lumen from the outside in, near the corner of one of the vessels (Fig. 47*B*). The suture then is carried to the opposite vessel and a horizontal mattress stitch is taken, *proceeding from the inside out and then from the outside in* (Fig. 47*C*). This technique is continued back and forth until the other corner is reached, at which point the suture is simply brought to the outside again by taking it from the inside out at the corner (Fig. 47*D*). This technical refinement is invaluable in performing critical venous anastomoses, such as end-to-side or side-to-side portasystemic shunts, or in venous anastomoses in organ transplantation, where exposure may be limited. In almost all other situations, continuous over-and-over sutures, proceeding to meet in the middle from each corner and with the most difficult corner or side sutured first, will provide the best and fastest anastomosis.

REMOVAL AND PREPARATION OF AUTOGRAFTS

The ideal graft replacement for an artery is another artery and for a vein, another vein. Ideally, these should also have identical dimensions. Clinical vascular surgery does not often offer such opportunities, however. The closest is the use of the hypogastric artery to perform aortorenal bypass in children. Fortunately, this artery is close to the correct size and can be removed unilaterally without serious consequences. Early in the "modern era" of vascular surgery, arterial homografts were explored with great enthusiasm, even to the point of freeze drying or lyophilizing them for long-term storage. Unfortunately, when implanted in a living host, degenerative and inflammatory changes soon ensued, resulting in aneurysm formation, mural calcification, and heightened susceptibility to atheromatous change. Saphenous vein homografts for peripheral arterial bypass have met with similar failure; that is, almost universal occlusion with time. Modified heterografts from several sources (e.g., bovine carotid artery and sheep connective tissue harvested after implanting mandrils) as well as human umbilical vein allografts have been tried, the latter having the greatest clinical success. Ficin digested to remove antigenic protein, wrapped in Dacron mesh to resist aneurysm formation, and stored in an aldehyde preservative, these grafts achieved roughly equivalent patency rates to that of the best available prosthesis (PTFE) in femorodistal bypass during the 1970s and early 1980s. Unfortunately, reports of late degenerative changes leading to aneurysm formation, in close to 50 percent in 5 years, have caused them to lose popularity. However, because of the disappointing results with small-caliber prosthetic grafts in infrageniculate bypass, interest in homografts has been rekindled, with research into ultraviolet radiation, better cryopreservation techniques, and other methods of preserving cellular integrity and viability and/or modifying antigenicity. Low-dose or short-course immunomodulation with newer drugs (such as SK 406) may ultimately serve as a useful adjunct, and entirely change the current perspective of vascular homografts.

Although these avenues all may hold some hope for the future, the focus here is on the methods that are practical and effective today, essentially limited to the use of superficial extremity vein autografts for extremity arterial bypass. The greater saphenous vein, in particular and, to a lesser extent, the lesser saphenous and cephalic veins have been extraordinarily useful in bypassing smaller arterial segments (i.e., less than 6 mm in diameter), the point beyond which the results with prosthetic grafts appear to worsen dramatically.

Saphenous vein autografts give unsurpassed patency rates in peripheral arterial bypass and are useful for renal, mesenteric, coronary, and carotid reconstructions. The vein's accessible superficial location and, because of the gravitational pressures in the lower extremities, its thicker wall make it a very suitable arterial substitute. It responds to arterial pressures with an increase in connective tissue and some loss of muscular elements. Though it loses some of its initial compliance, the retention (or restitution) of an endothelial surface is largely responsible for its unparalleled performance as an arterial bypass graft, with 5-year patency rates close to 80 percent now being achieved.

Because of availability and proven performance, these vein autografts are employed whenever possible for the longer (i.e., infrageniculate) leg bypasses and even shorter bypasses to smaller distal arteries. Their frequent use and the clear importance of proper removal and preparation in achieving their potential justify the focus on the technique of vein "harvest" here under basic techniques. It is an essential component of many, if not most, peripheral arterial bypasses.

The location of the saphenous or cephalic veins may be apparent by inspection of thin patients or by reference to anatomy books, and the location of their origins and terminations is quite reliable. However, variations in anatomy between these points are not uncommon (about 25 percent), and these, or prior injury or phlebitic occlusion of intervening segments, may not be apparent from casual inspection. Therefore, the author prefers to have the patency, diameter, and anatomic course of prospective venous autografts directly assessed by duplex scanning before all elective operations. Mapping these details on the overlying skin with indelible marking is extremely helpful, particularly in patients whose superficial veins have been partly or completely removed by stripping for varicosities or for previous bypass. In such cases, duplex scanning often reveals compensatory enlargement of the ipsilateral lesser saphenous vein, a usable residual segment of ipsilateral greater saphenous, or an adequate contralateral saphenous vein. Segmental diameter measurements help determine the most appropriate segment and whether or not reversal or antegrade placement after valvulotomy is most appropriate.

Although two- or three-step incisions over the course of the greater saphenous vein may allow more cosmetic removal during femoropopliteal bypass, most surgeons agree that direct exposure by a single overlying longitudinal incision allows less traumatic removal and that is an overriding consideration. Other considerations may come into play for obtaining short segments of vein graft for patch angioplasty or short interposition graft. The best vein is ordinarily the greater saphenous, followed by the lesser saphenous, lower cephalic, and basilic veins, in that order. The upper greater saphenous vein is larger and thick-walled but more deeply located than it is distally. The vein has larger but less frequent tributaries and fewer valves per unit length. Furthermore, the author has found better preservation of patency and diameter in the residual vein following proximal rather than distal *partial* removal. Still, preservation of the proximal greater

Basic Vascular Techniques

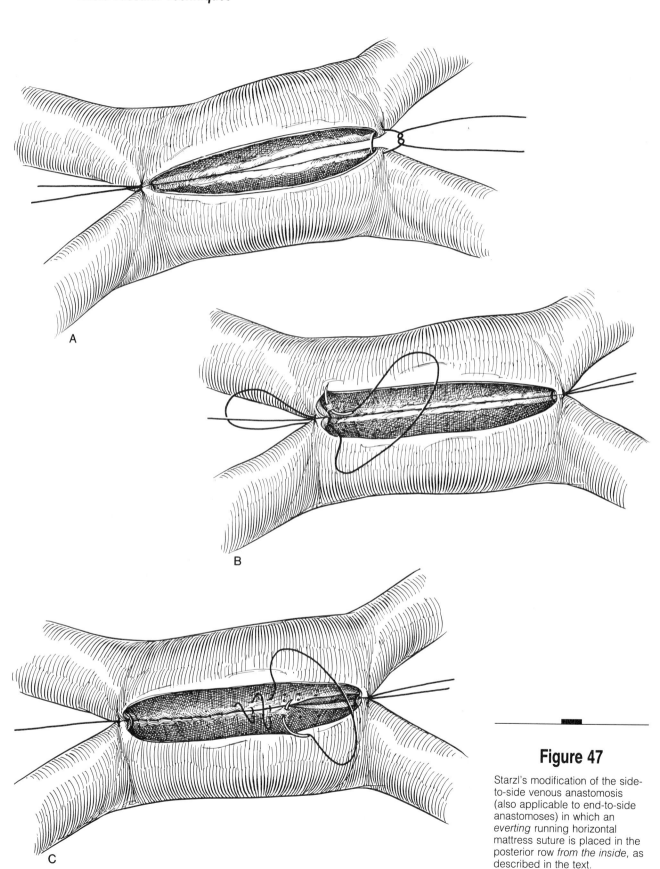

A

B

C

Figure 47

Starzl's modification of the side-to-side venous anastomosis (also applicable to end-to-side anastomoses) in which an *everting* running horizontal mattress suture is placed in the posterior row *from the inside*, as described in the text.

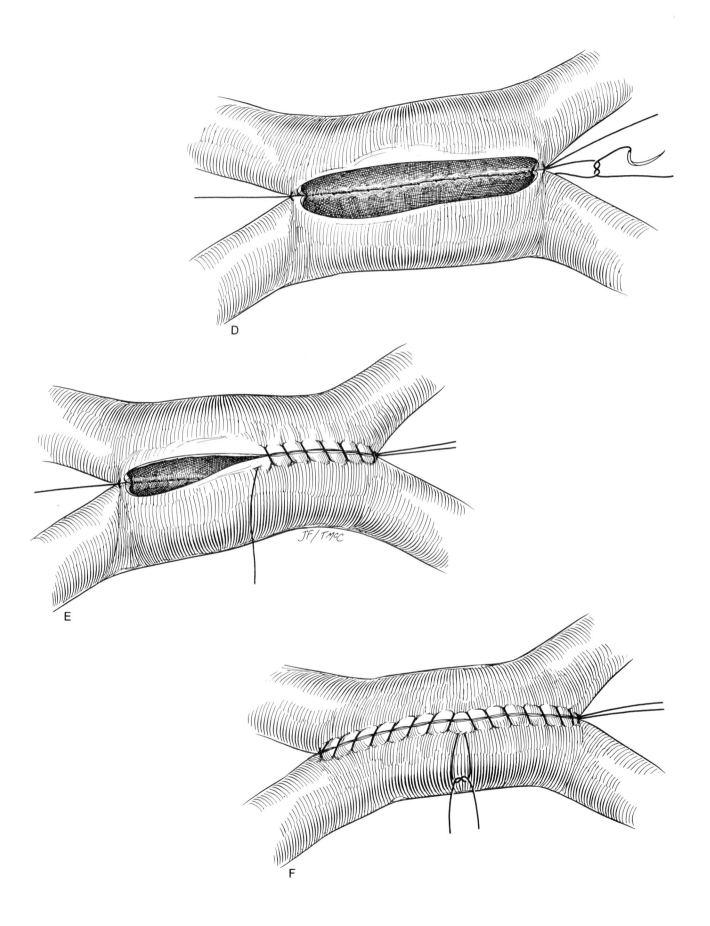

D

E

F

Basic Vascular Techniques

saphenous holds the greatest future value should femorodistal bypass become necessary, making this an overriding consideration.

Vein harvest is best performed by incising the skin directly over the course of the vein to be removed and exposing its anterior surface along the entire length required before beginning actual removal. In this regard, once the vein has been exposed at either end, because there are no directly anterior branches, the fastest, safest, and most accurate method of progressive exposure is by repeatedly sliding the tips of a scissors or long clamp (e.g., a tonsil clamp) along the course of the next most adjacent venous segment and incising over the spread tips, which are lifted upward protecting the underlying vein from injury (Fig. 48*A*).

The exposed vein must be kept moist by frequently bathing it with physiologic salt solution. The addition of papaverine (at 60 mg per liter) to this solution is helpful in preventing venospasm. Gently infiltrating small amounts of this solution around the vein before proceeding with its removal is also recommended, for persistent spasm almost guarantees loss of the endothelial surface, which requires 2 weeks to be restored under the best of conditions. Next, beginning at one end, a Silastic loop is placed under the vein. Gentle upward traction lifts the vein from its bed and, by placing entering tributaries under tension, identifies their location (Fig. 48*B*). These are ligated 1 mm from their point of entry with from 2-0 to 4-0 silk ligatures, depending on their caliber. The distal ends are ligated or clipped before division. The surrounding tissue is sharply dissected away with Metzenbaum scissors, leaving 2 to 3 mm of tissue around the vein (Fig. 48*C*). Not only does this buffer it from the harmful effects of directly baring its surface but also, if any small unseen tributaries are transected at this distance from the surface, they will still have a sufficient residual cuff to allow easy ligation later. As the vein is freed from its bed, the Silastic loop is slid along to aid in its exposure. Flow is allowed to continue through the vein until it has been completely exposed and is ready for removal. Then, the vein is ligated distally and cannulated and flushed before proximal ligation and division. The irrigating solution preferred by the author is Dextran 40 with 30 mg of papaverine and 500 units of heparin added to each 500-ml unit. This solution is cooled to 4°C only if the vein will *not* be implanted immediately.

A large (30- to 50-ml) syringe is attached to the cannula with a three-way stopcock interposed and with the operator's other fingers pinching the vein lumen at increasing distances from the cannulated end. Thus, sequential segments of the vein are gently dilated and checked for leaks (Fig. 49). The large syringe makes it less likely that physiologic pressures will be exceeded. Peak pressures should be kept between 120 and 200 mmHg, roughly equivalent to the range of arterial pressures the vein will be subjected to in the leg in the recumbent and standing positions, respectively. Small branches cut with a 2-mm stump can easily be clamped and tied if visualized while the irrigant is still spurting from its end (Fig. 49*A*). The orifices of accidentally avulsed branches should be accurately oversewn with 7-0 polypropylene suture, preferably under magnification, while a stream of irrigating solution not only allows one to visualize its exact location but also holds it open in an expanded position (Fig. 49*B*). A carefully harvested vein should have few if any such leaks.

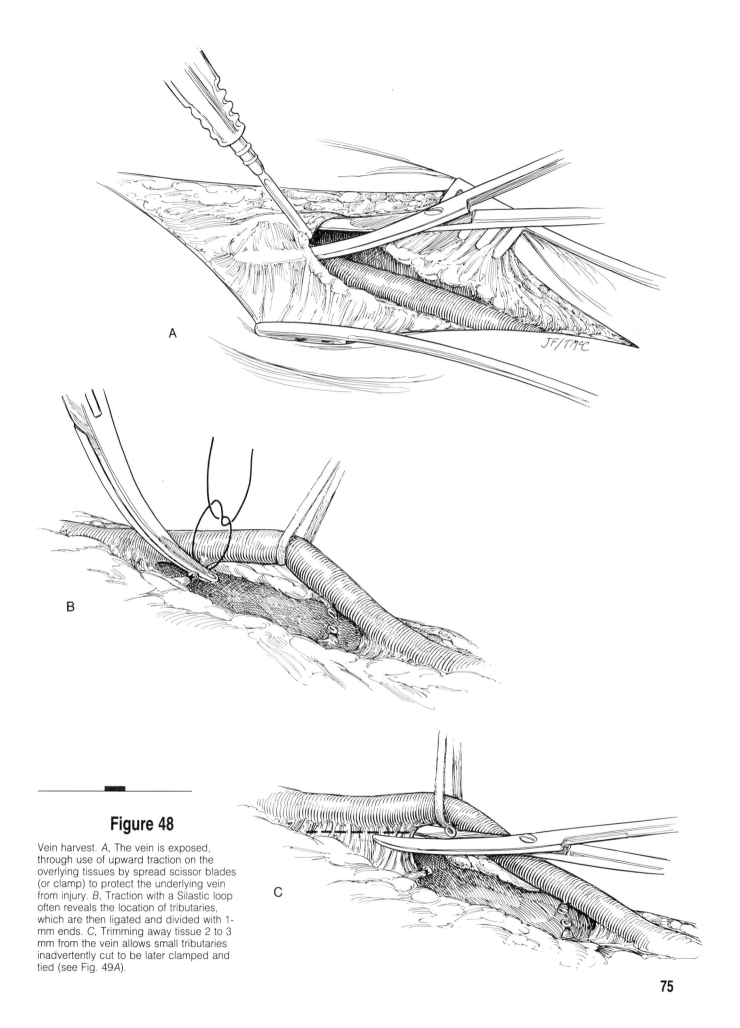

Figure 48

Vein harvest. *A*, The vein is exposed, through use of upward traction on the overlying tissues by spread scissor blades (or clamp) to protect the underlying vein from injury. *B*, Traction with a Silastic loop often reveals the location of tributaries, which are then ligated and divided with 1-mm ends. *C*, Trimming away tissue 2 to 3 mm from the vein allows small tributaries inadvertently cut to be later clamped and tied (see Fig. 49*A*).

Basic Vascular Techniques

This process having been completed, the vein is now ready for use in a reversed anatomic (not flow) orientation as an arterial bypass graft. In this reversed orientation, the vein valves offer little resistance to flow. However, if the caliber of the vein tapers too much over its length, a "diameter mismatch" may be created by this reverse orientation. Thus, in a typical femorotibial bypass, one may find oneself anastomosing the small end (i.e., 3-mm internal diameter, ID) of the saphenous vein into the much larger femoral arterial segment proximally (6- to 8-mm ID), then sewing the larger end of the vein (5- to 6-mm ID) into a much smaller tibial artery (2-mm ID) distally.

Therefore, if it is not feasible to perform this bypass in situ, it is the author's preference to take advantage of valvulotomy techniques. These were developed for in situ bypass to render the valves incompetent. Their use here allows the vein autograft to be *translocated* and used in an orthograde orientation, which provides a more suitable matching of dimensions at each anastomosis. The particular valvulotome chosen for this or the in situ technique itself is, to some extent, a matter of personal preference. Some of the available options are shown in Figure 50. The first valve or two at the upper end are better cut with valvulotomy scissors (Fig. 50A). Once this is done, the valve cutter of choice or its stem can be introduced from below into the prepared upper segment. At this point, it is best to distend the vein using infusate introduced from above. With the Leather valve cutter (Fig. 50B), the infusion catheter is drawn along with it by a linking suture, distending each new segment before the next valve is cut. With a Hall or LeMaitre valvulotome or similar modifications of appropriate size (Fig. 50D), the upper end may be cannulated and distended with infusate before valvulotome withdrawal. At the distal end, if the vein tapers down in caliber even the smaller-sized of the aforementioned valvulotomes may be too large. Here, a thin Mills valvulotome may be introduced from below, to cut each of the lower valve cusps (Fig. 50C). The vein can be telescoped over it to allow it to reach higher or it can be introduced through side branches. Mehigan has popularized an effective use of an angioscope to facilitate valvulotomy. The angioscope advances down the vein and monitors the application of the valvulotome, as shown for a specially lengthened Mills-type valvulotome in Figure 50C; in addition, its infusion port allows segmental venous distension during the procedure. The additional advantages of this approach include not only the setting up of the valve cusp for accurate cutting and the relative lack of contact between valvulotome and the endothelialized inner surface of the vein afforded by the vein distention, but also the visualization of each cut valve and each major deep venous connection. By stopping the angioscope at these major deep branches, the overlying skin may be marked where it is transilluminated by the lighted head of the angioscope for later reference. In performing all of these valve cutting maneuvers, remember that the cusps of the valves of superficial veins meet in a plane *parallel* with the overlying skin. The cutting edge of many of the available valvulotome instruments, therefore, must be kept perpendicular to this. One warning pertains to the common location of branches just distal to cusps. These can be inadvertently caught by a valvulotome and the vein torn at this point because the resistance they offer is mistaken for a valve cusp or they are caught in the "backlash" of cutting the adjacent valve. Correct sizing of the valvulotome and distension of the vein wall when cutting will help prevent these injuries.

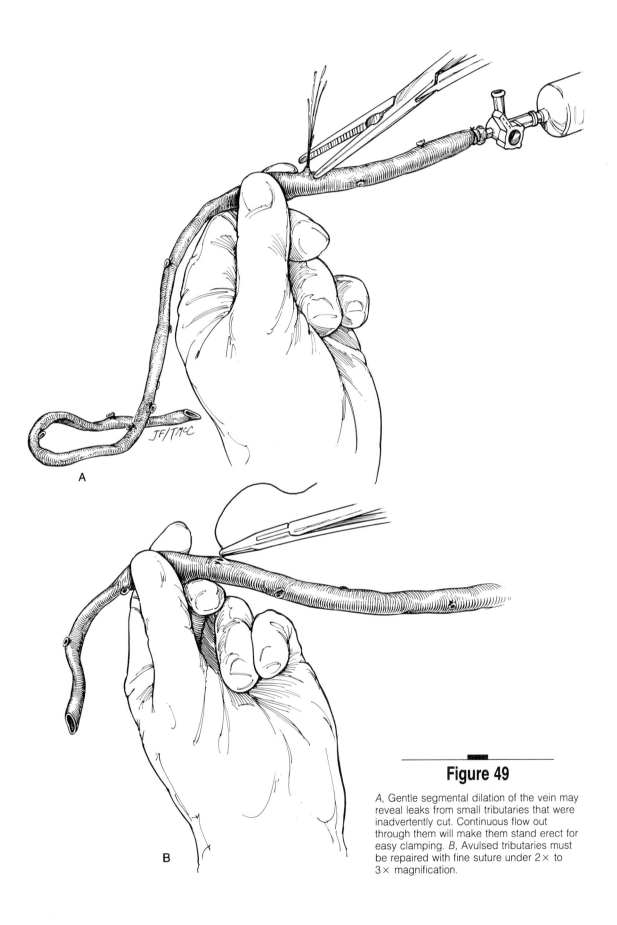

A

B

Figure 49

A, Gentle segmental dilation of the vein may reveal leaks from small tributaries that were inadvertently cut. Continuous flow out through them will make them stand erect for easy clamping. *B*, Avulsed tributaries must be repaired with fine suture under 2× to 3× magnification.

Basic Vascular Techniques

TUNNELING

Most peripheral arterial bypasses employ a conduit that joins patent segments above and below the obstructing lesions, by end-to-side anastomosis at each end. The site of the proximal and distal anastomoses is often selected as much for ease of access and familiarity with exposure as for freedom from disease. An essential step in this process is passage of the graft through an appropriate anatomic pathway between these two incisions, commonly called tunneling. The appropriate anatomic pathway for each bypass differs and is discussed separately for each such procedure. The basic tunneling sequence is the same and is described here.

The first and simplest is shown in Figure 51, employing femorofemoral bypass as the prototype. If the two incisions are relatively close or the operator's fingers are long, or both, one can create a tunnel; pass a long instrument, such as a slightly curved DeBakey aneurysm clamp through it; and pull an umbilical tape or a Penrose drain back again. This serves as a marker to relocate the passage when the time comes to pass the graft through it. Later, when the clamp is reintroduced into the tunnel, it should grasp the end of the tape or drain and be pulled, not pushed, through the same passage. The reason this is not done at the same time is that tunneling is preferred *before* heparin is given, and graft passage is often performed *after* the first anastomosis, when the patient is fully heparinized. If a Penrose drain is placed, the tip of the clamp can be slid *inside* the end of the drain, grasping an inward fold of the thin, pliable latex rubber, thereby allowing it to be drawn through the tunnel without catching on any tissue or structure (Fig. 51*C*).

For longer or unusually curved tunnels, a number of special instruments called tunnelers are available to facilitate this part of the procedure. One of them is depicted in Figure 52*A* through *F* to illustrate the proper sequence. The tunneling is begun in the correct plane from either end using the index fingers *(A)*. Then, the tunneler is introduced into one end, advanced along the proper pathway toward the waiting finger at the other end *(B)*. After proper passage, the rounded tip of the device is removed *(C)* and the graft is firmly attached to it by suture ligature so that axial rotation is impossible *(D)*. Most modern prostheses have linear orientation marks, but vein grafts must be oriented by careful inspection before the correct axial orientation is determined and maintained by finger grasp of the tip. The graft is then drawn back through the outer sheath by withdrawing the inner obturator while maintaining finger grasp on the (previously oriented) other end. The leading tip of the graft is brought up to, but not through, the far end of the tunneler sheath *(E)*. A common mistake is to deliver it there and cut off the attached tip. Orientation can potentially be lost when the sheath is withdrawn over the graft. Instead, the sheath should be withdrawn in the same direction back onto the obturator, exposing the properly oriented forward tip of the graft, as it exits from the other wound *(F)*. Then, it may be securely grasped *before* the tip is cut off so that one is certain it lies properly oriented in the tunnel. Before proceeding with the first anastomosis, the graft at the other end should be clamped in such a way (also incorporating tissue, drapes, or tapes) that the orienting clamp cannot be displaced and inadvertently rotated 360°.

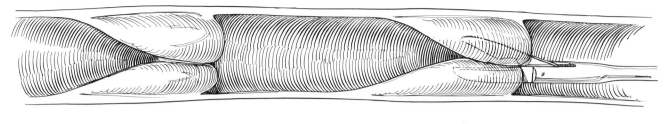

A

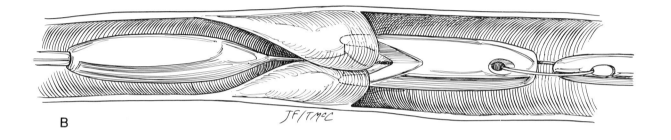

B

JF/TMcC

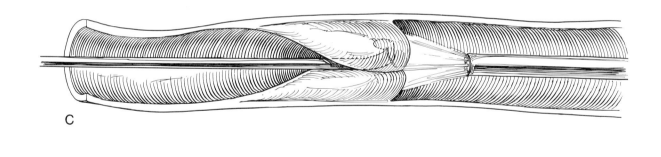

C

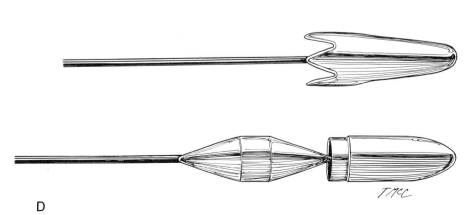

Figure 50

Some valvulotomy instruments and techniques. *A,* Cutting the upper valve with a valvulotome scissors. *B,* Passage of the Leather valve cutter linked by suture to a 5F irrigating catheter to distend the lumen. *C,* Cutting each valve cuff with a Mills valvulotome, here under direct angioscopic surveillance. *D,* An assortment of metal valvulotomes including the Hall (above) and the LeMaitre (below). In the middle is a modified valvulotome with a slightly in-curving, scalloped cutting edge, provided by Jao Carlos Palazzo, a vascular surgeon in Rio de Janeiro.

D

TMcC

Basic Vascular Techniques

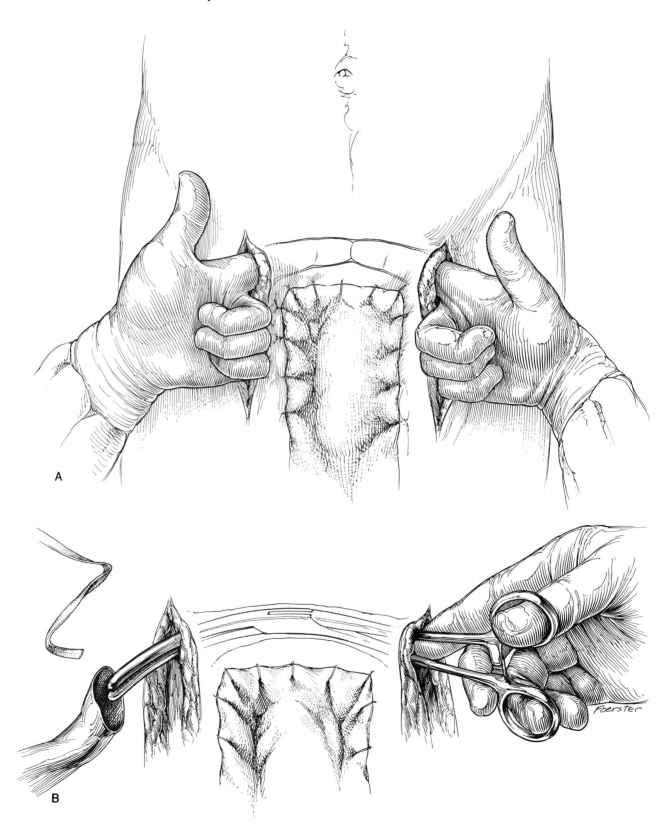

A

B

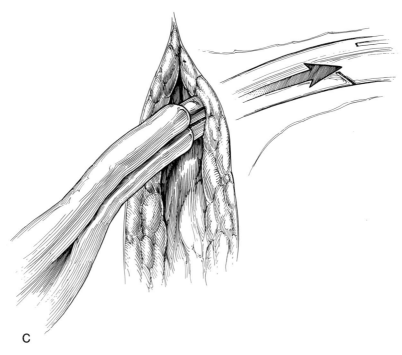

C

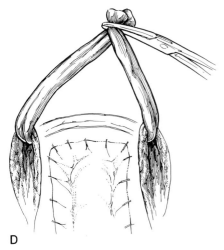

D

Figure 51

A, Simple finger tunneling between two reasonably close incisions (here shown for femorofemoral bypass). B, Passage of a long curved clamp to grasp an umbilical tape or Penrose drain. C, Grasping an *inside* edge of the drain allows easy passage in either direction. D, Clamping the drain ends until needed later. E, Withdrawal of the clamp back through the tunnel to accept the graft.

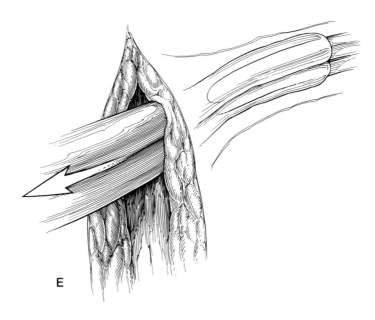

E

Basic Vascular Techniques

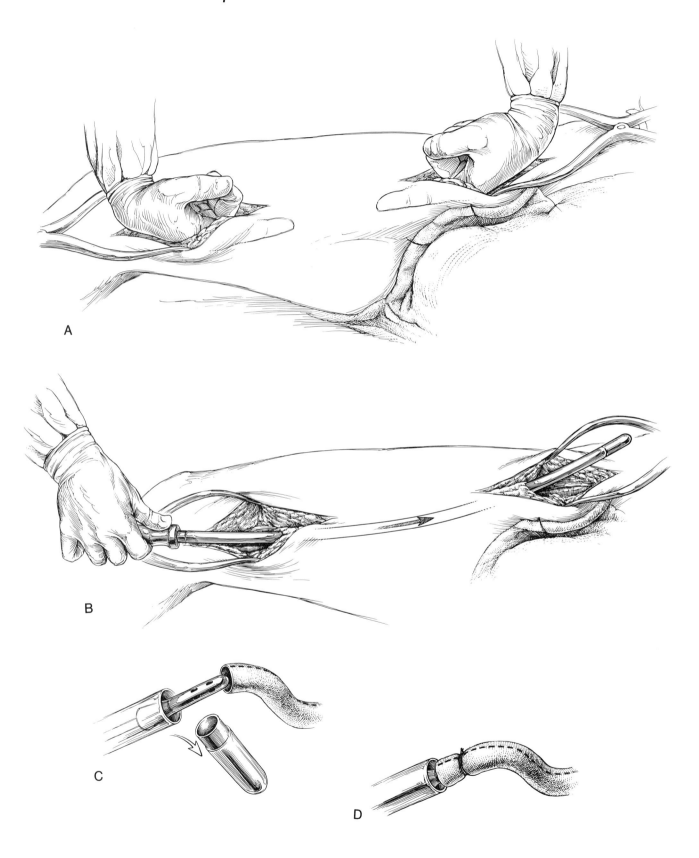

A

B

C

D

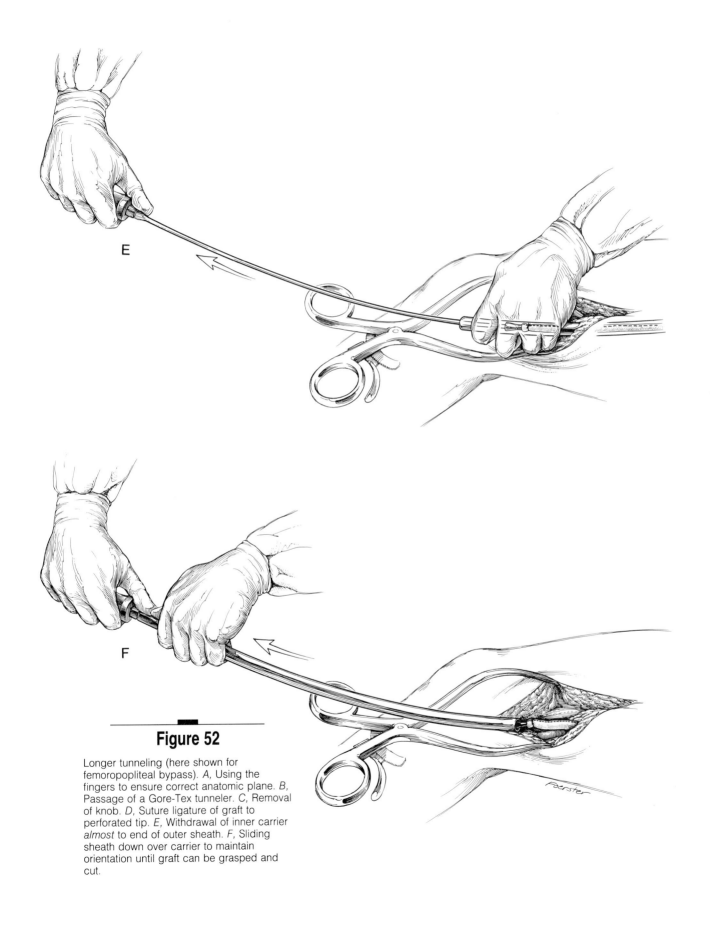

Figure 52

Longer tunneling (here shown for femoropopliteal bypass). *A*, Using the fingers to ensure correct anatomic plane. *B*, Passage of a Gore-Tex tunneler. *C*, Removal of knob. *D*, Suture ligature of graft to perforated tip. *E*, Withdrawal of inner carrier *almost* to end of outer sheath. *F*, Sliding sheath down over carrier to maintain orientation until graft can be grasped and cut.

THROMBOEMBOLECTOMY AND OTHER USES OF FOGARTY BALLOON CATHETERS

Before the introduction of balloon catheter embolectomy by Thomas Fogarty in 1963, there was no satisfactory way of removing luminal thrombus. Long forceps, doubled strands of stiff stainless steel wire with a "ski-tip" upward bend at the end, and long thin suction catheters had all been used but were quickly put aside with the arrival of balloon catheters. Like many great inventions, both the design and operating principle are elegantly simple. Thin-walled balloons of different sizes are attached to the tips of long thin hollow catheters similar in consistency to ureteral catheters and having similar markings for gauging distances. They are inflated through the hollow catheter by a syringe attached to the hub, with or without an intervening three-way stopcock (Fig. 53). After gaining control of the vessel to be entered, they are introduced through an arteriotomy or a venotomy, passed beyond the clot, inflated, and withdrawn, thereby extracting the clot (Fig. 54*A* through *C*). Thus, the Fogarty balloon catheter is elegantly simple in principle, yet many small details of execution are critical to its success and to avoiding vascular injury.

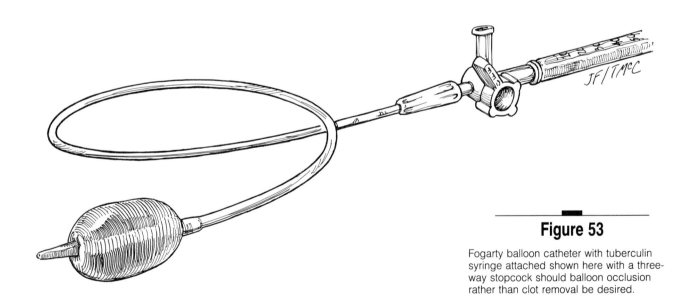

Figure 53

Fogarty balloon catheter with tuberculin syringe attached shown here with a three-way stopcock should balloon occlusion rather than clot removal be desired.

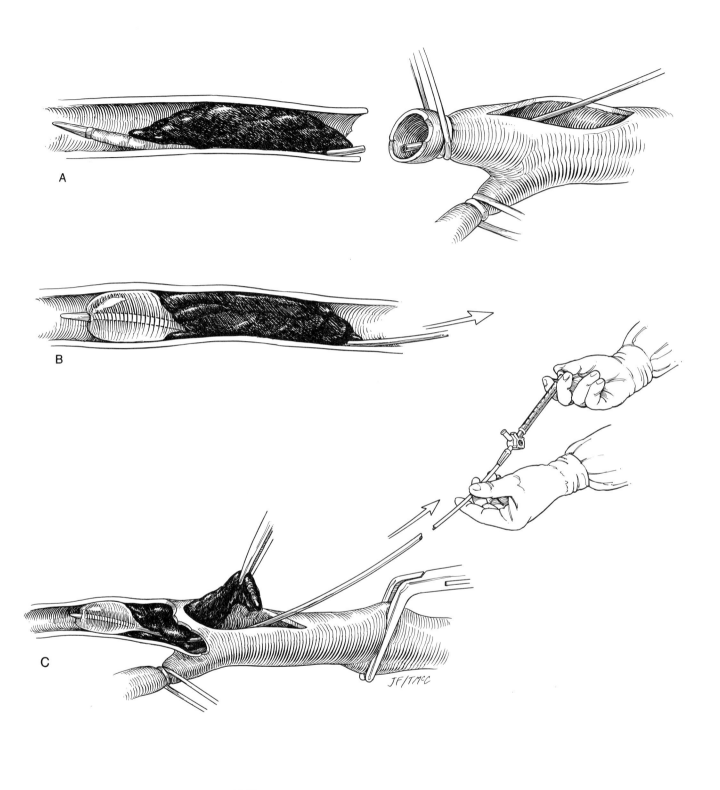

Figure 54

Basic technique of thromboembolectomy
using a Fogarty balloon catheter with
insertion beyond the clot *(A)*, inflation *(B)*,
and withdrawal *(C)*.

Basic Vascular Techniques

Arterial embolectomy catheters have a firmer tip and run from 1F to 6F. Venous thrombectomy catheters have a softer, more flexible tip designed to negotiate venous valves when passed distally and reach up to a 10F size. The 1F catheter is inflated with air; the others with saline in volumes from 0.2 ml upward, as indicated on the catheter, using 1-ml and 3-ml syringes as needed. After inflating and deflating the catheter and balloon to ensure against leaks or eccentric inflation and to fill the catheter dead space with saline, the recommended filling volume should be strictly adhered to and not exceeded. Connections with the syringe must be wetted and be securely air tight. Several test inflations ensure consistent inflation and pliability.

The catheter should be placed on the patient proximally and distally from the point of vessel entry to gauge approximate distances to key anatomic landmarks. For example, from a femoral arteriotomy it may be 20 cm up to the aortic bifurcation, 45 cm down to the popliteal trifurcation, and 65 to 70 cm to the ankle. This distance may be important in localizing occlusive lesions or other restrictions of catheter advancement or withdrawal. After wetting the deflated tip, the catheter is introduced distally up to a predetermined distance. Meeting early resistance may mean one has encountered organized thrombus; the embolus may have occurred within hours, but its constituent thrombus material may have been forming at the proximal site of origin for weeks or months! Possibly, one may have inadvertently entered a collateral branch; for example, if the profunda femoris has been entered, the catheter will stop at 20 to 25 cm. Conversely, there may have been a false passage or a preexisting occlusive lesion that has blocked catheter passage. After backing up and reintroducing the catheter, if the same obstruction is repeatedly met at the same point, the operator should back up the catheter a centimeter, gently inflate the balloon until the first feeling of resistance is met, and withdraw it. Removal of a small amount of organized thrombus should facilitate further attempts at passage. Repeated incomplete passages dictate angiographic or angioscopic investigation.

Ordinarily, recent embolus or propagated thrombus is easily passed by the catheter tip and one proceeds to the predetermined distance for full insertion. If one were performing a distal thromboembolectomy through an incision in the common femoral artery, one would likely then be in either the distal peroneal artery or the posterior tibial artery, for the anterior tibial artery is difficult to enter deliberately unless the tibioperoneal trunk has been chronically occluded. The balloon is then gently and only *partially* inflated in this smaller artery, until traction on it produces the first feel of contact but not "drag." This is an important difference in sensation, which comes to most surgeons only with experience. To sense this properly, it is important to have the same person pulling on the catheter with one hand while controlling inflation with the other.

During withdrawal, as one enters the distal popliteal artery, a significant adjustment in the degree of inflation will have to be made and thereafter minor adjustments will be needed, as the caliber of the tapered proximal artery increases. Catheter returns should not simply be suctioned away but should be carefully inspected and, if warranted, sent for histologic examination to rule out myxoma or determine the age and dominant component of the clot or even sent for culture. Brisk backflow may or *may not* signal success. Two subsequent negative passes and completion angioscopy or angiography are necessary before declaring success.

Proximal passage will require reverse adjustments in balloon inflation to accommodate decreasing vessel caliber on withdrawal. Passage upward, above the aortic bifurcation, and full inflation of a larger (i.e., 5F to 6F) catheter will allow it to hang up at the common iliac orifice as it is withdrawn, after which sequential deflations will allow safe extraction of iliac clot. Saddle emboli are approached via bilateral femoral incisions. Transverse arteriotomy incisions are preferred if one is sure one is dealing with acute embolism and not chronic occlusive disease with secondary thrombosis. In the latter instance, a longitudinal arteriotomy is preferable because it may serve as the site of a proximal bypass anastomosis.

Fogarty balloon catheters are not yet guidable and thus tend to enter only one and the same infrapopliteal branch with distal passage from a common femoral arteriotomy. Knee flexion, placing a second catheter down while the first is still in place, and bending the catheter tip may or may not succeed in overcoming this impasse. If angioscopy or angiography confirms incomplete clot removal, distal instillation of 250,000 units of urokinase for 20 to 30 minutes, followed by distal irrigation and additional balloon catheter passes, may produce an acceptable end result. If not, the author prefers exploring the origins of the infrapopliteal branches through the standard medial below-knee popliteal exposure (see Section 2) and placing a transverse arteriotomy in the distal popliteal artery just proximal to the anterior tibial artery orifice so that the latter artery, as well as the peroneal and posterior tibial arteries, may each be selectively entered and disobliterated.

Venous thrombectomy requires larger catheters, even gentler technique, and negotiation of distal valves. Whenever possible, the author prefers to minimize the inevitable endothelial damage from the balloon catheter by applying sequential external compression to extrude the distal clot *without using a balloon catheter.* This is best done by manual external massage, tight wrapping of an Esmarch bandage, repeat foot dorsiflexions, or their combination. If the thrombus is recent, it can regularly remove distal clot without *any* catheter thrombectomy, thereby minimizing intimal damage that promotes rethrombosis. A catheter passed proximally for embolectomy does not encounter any valves but may be misdirected up the ascending lumbar vein, or one may have difficulty passing iliac artery compression on the left. Therefore, completion venography in the proximal direction is mandatory to ensure full iliac vein patency with no extrinsic or intrinsic obstruction.

Basic Vascular Techniques

Vascular Control by Balloon Occlusion. Major branches or distal arteries may be better controlled from within the lumen using gentle balloon occlusion, held in place by closure of a three-way stopcock. A good example of this application is when the profunda femoris is deeply placed and obscured by scar tissue or located somewhere on the posterior surface of a large femoral pseudoaneurysm, which is adherent to the adjacent vein or has splayed out the femoral nerve. Rather than a tedious or dangerous dissection to expose and loop the origin of the profunda femoris artery, one needs only to gain proximal and distal control of the common and superficial femoral arteries, respectively, and then control the profunda femoris through the arteriotomy with a balloon catheter (Fig. 55). This approach also works well if one wishes to avoid placing a vascular clamp across a heavily calcified distal artery during bypass or to control an inaccessible distal internal carotid artery when the proximal vessel is involved with aneurysm or penetrating trauma. In the former circumstance (usually peroneal or tibial bypass in diabetic patients), however, the use of a sterile tourniquet, as advocated by Bernhard and Towne, has much to recommend it.

Aberrant renal arteries, encountered unexpectedly during aortic aneurysm repair, can also be readily controlled by small balloon catheter inflation. Occasionally, when irreparable damage to an artery has occurred or when irradiation and scar tissue combine to prevent safe dissection and suture closure, balloon catheters can be inserted and left in place for several days until occlusion by accumulating thrombus is reliably firm and attached. Then sequential deflation over several days will allow safe withdrawal. Acquired arteriovenous fistulas, difficult to approach because of an overlying network of tense veins, may be occluded and controlled by advancing a balloon catheter via an accessible arteriotomy site located proximally or distally and gently inflating and withdrawing it until the palpable thrill, or continuous high-velocity sound heard with a Doppler, ceases. The fistula may then be more safely approached. This approach is now feasible in some locations by percutaneously inserted catheters employing detachable balloons.

Larger Fogarty balloons (e.g., 8–22F) are available for aortic occlusion and are useful in ruptured abdominal aortic aneurysm, major abdominal vascular injury, secondary aortoenteric fistulas, or, for that matter, any aortic bleeding from a site not readily accessible because of location or surrounding adhesions or scarring. Placed through a transverse arteriotomy in the mid-brachial artery, the catheter should first be measured to gauge approximate distances to the aortic arch and to the juxtarenal aorta. Once inserted to the former distance, its location in the aorta can be confirmed by one's ability to inflate it fully. It should then be partially deflated and withdrawn, until it engages the subclavian orifice before being gently advanced again. This time it will be drawn downward by the forceful aortic pulsations against the partially inflated balloon. Once in place, the balloon may be either immediately and fully inflated, as in the rapidly deteriorating patient, or left deflated until needed during a difficult direct dissection to gain control. The latter approach minimizes suprarenal occlusion time. Similar large catheters, such as a 16F 30-cc balloon Foley catheter, can be introduced up the aorta and later down into the iliac arteries via the rent in a bleeding aortic aneurysm, if rapid dissection of the neck of the aneurysm is not feasible.

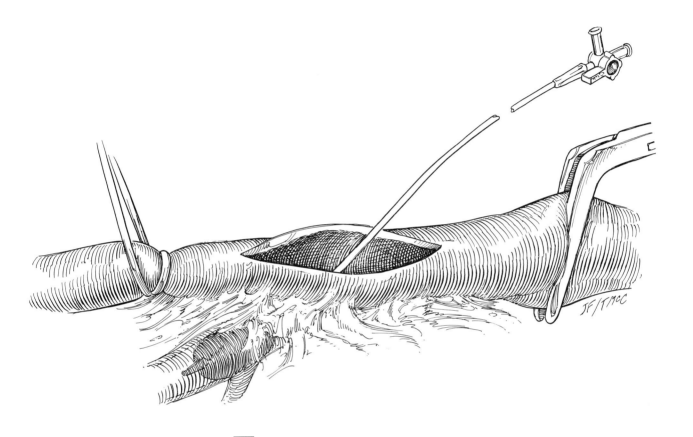

Figure 55

Use of the Fogarty balloon catheter for
controlled occlusion of major branch. (Here
the profunda femoris artery is obscured by
scar tissue.)

Basic Vascular Techniques

ENDARTERECTOMY

In the over four decades since its introduction by Dos Santos, and subsequent popularization in the United States by Wylie, endarterectomy has waxed and waned in popularity. In the author's view, it still can play a significant role, not only as the preferred technique for atheromatous disease at the carotid bifurcation but also, *when selectively applied,* as the principal procedure at other major sites (e.g., aortoiliac endarterectomy, femoral profundaplasty). Furthermore, it may be used to advantage as an adjunctive procedure to bypass grafting at both the inflow and outflow ends and to manage orificial disease involving major aortic branches. It is interesting that at a time when many vascular surgeons in their own practices have essentially limited endarterectomy to the carotid bifurcation, many others are greeting much cruder forms of endovascular obliteration, by laser ablation and atherectomy devices, with enthusiasm. It is doubtful that any of these techniques will ever produce as "clean" a removal of the obstructing atheromatous process as does endarterectomy. The predictable lack of durability of these newer endovascular procedures appears to have been taken lightly only because of the relatively minor entry site through which they can be performed.

Endarterectomy takes advantage of a natural cleavage plane that develops in the outer media of aging arteries, the same one that is so readily followed during a spontaneous arterial dissection. Atherosclerotic plaque formation ordinarily involves only the inner arterial wall (i.e., the intima and some of the media), stopping short of the usual depth of endarterectomy. Unless there has already been aneurysmal degeneration, the outer myoelastic layers of the media, the external elastic lamellae, and the adventitia are healthy and strong enough to resist aneurysm development. After endarterectomy and re-endothelialization of the healed inner surface, the remaining layers serve as a durable arterial conduit. Preexisting aneurysmal degeneration is the only absolute categoric contraindication to endarterectomy. Control of the sometimes exuberant healing process, which may lead to neointimal hyperplasia and restenosis, is almost the only thing that stands in the way of a uniformly excellent outcome. However, when the disease is extensive rather than discrete, a complete endarterectomy is difficult to perform and restenosis is not uncommon.

Endarterectomy is a single method of disobliteration, which can be accomplished by a number of different techniques that can be employed singly or in combination. In *open* endarterectomy, the segmental plaque is completely exposed by a longitudinal arteriotomy and removed under direct vision. This approach is commonly applied in carotid and aortoiliac endarterectomy and, depending on the residual lumen, may or may not be closed with a patch. More often the open technique is modified at one or the other end or at a major branch by employing *eversion, semiclosed,* or *orificial* endarterectomy. All these techniques are illustrated in the generic description of endarterectomy that follows, one that might be applied to atheromatous disease at a major arterial bifurcation (e.g., femoral, carotid, iliac).

A longitudinal incision is made along the superior surface of the common arterial trunk from the level of palpable plaque proximally to a short way into one or the other of the two main outflow vessels, depending on the distribution of palpable disease and the relative importance of restoring outflow to each (Fig. 56). If both are equally important or if there is significant disease in both that seems amenable to these techniques, one may direct the incision toward the

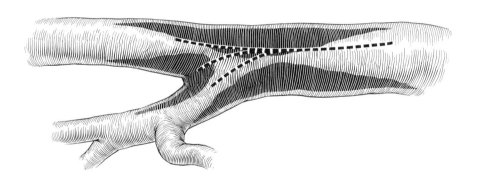

Figure 56

Longitudinal incision for endarterectomy with optimal extensions based on knowledge or palpation of extent of underlying disease.

Basic Vascular Techniques

bifurcation between them. Ordinarily, however, it is directed along the most critical outflow vessel with an awareness to the possible need for extension.

The incision is made gently down to the aforementioned cleavage plane, shown in a cross-sectional view in Figure 57. This is usually easily seen and may be developed circumferentially without entering the lumen, particularly when the plaque obliterates most of the lumen. However, in most cases, the disease is eccentric with the least involved part of the circumference directly accessible from the superior aspect. When one can palpate this soft anterior wall, it should be entered and completely opened at the time of the initial arteriotomy. Inspecting or teasing of the cut edge of the arterial wall will reveal the appropriate cleavage plane in the outer media (Fig. 58A). Usually, the two layers will readily split apart at this point and, using the blade of a Penfield or Freer dissector, this plane is easily separated circumferentially (Fig. 58B). In some instances, the entire plaque can be removed in one piece. In other cases, a right-angle clamp is passed underneath the plaque by gently pushing and spreading in this plane posteriorly to join the two sides of the dissection, and the specimen then can be divided over this (Fig. 58C). By grasping each half, one can proceed toward each end with the advantage of being able to dissect circumferentially under direct vision, using traction on the specimen to great advantage (Fig. 58D).

Usually, one performs the least critical ends of the endarterectomy first, trimming off the proximal end point (Fig. 58E), then the minor branch (Fig. 58D), and finally the major or most critical outflow vessel. The goal is to obtain a smooth tapering separation of the specimen at the distal end points just beyond the natural tapering of the atheromatous plaque, leaving a thin adherent edge of relatively normal intima. When the plaque formation ends a short distance into the arterial branch, it may be separated by gently inserting the Penfield dissector along one aspect of the circumference of the plaque. After breaking through into the lumen at a natural end point, one repeats this process circumferentially using lateral as well as longitudinal stroking motions while applying countertraction to the specimen to separate off this branch extension of the plaque (Fig. 58D).

It is a natural extension of this technique, by applying persistent, even traction on the specimen, to produce an *eversion* of the outer wall (Fig. 59). One can more easily employ the spatulated blade of the endarterectomy instrument to develop this plane and extract the specimen of inner plaque from the outer arterial wall, as it progressively turns inside out (Fig. 59A and B). When the natural end point is reached, the steady traction usually makes the specimen separate cleanly, with an evenly tapered termination which, for reasons unknown to the author, has been termed "feathering." Seeing this thin, almost translucent edge provides evidence of a satisfactory end point. This should be confirmed by inspection, irrigating through a fine cannula tip to see if a loose intimal flap remains that will be lifted up by a jet of fluid coming in that direction. If this is the case, or the residual intima of the end point is obviously still thick, the arteriotomy should be open to just beyond this point, the remaining protruding edge of the inner layer trimmed flush and the edge secured to the outer wall by a number of end-on, through-and-through fine monofilament sutures tied on the outside.

Figure 60 shows the rationale behind this maneuver. When the flow is restored in the presence of such a loose intimal edge, the pulsatile force of arterial flow will progressively insinuate itself under this and dissect it upward and inward until it curls in and occludes the lumen (Fig. 60*A* and *B*). This can be prevented by the described "tack-down" sutures shown in horizontal and cross section in Figure 60*C* and *D*. If the outflow vessel is of small diameter, narrowing at this tack-down site can be obviated by patch closure, provided the tip of the patch reaches *beyond this point.*

Text continued on page 98

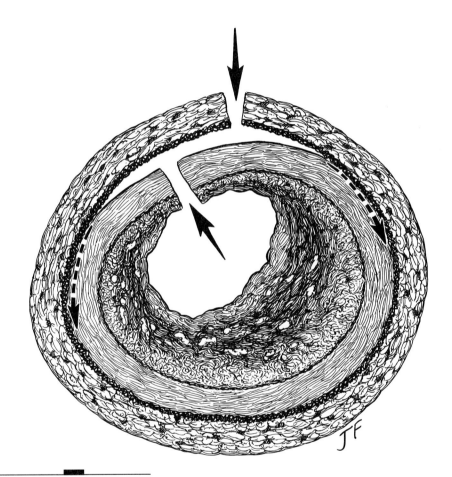

Figure 57

Cross section of a diseased artery showing incision to the correct level (cleavage plane in outer media), which is then followed circumferentially.

Basic Vascular Techniques

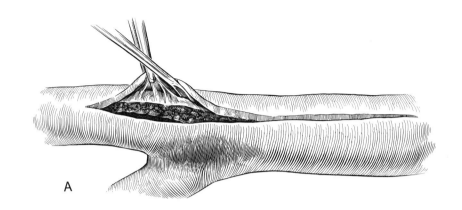

A

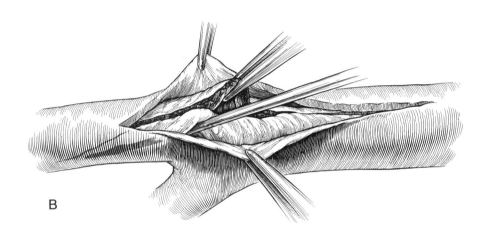

B

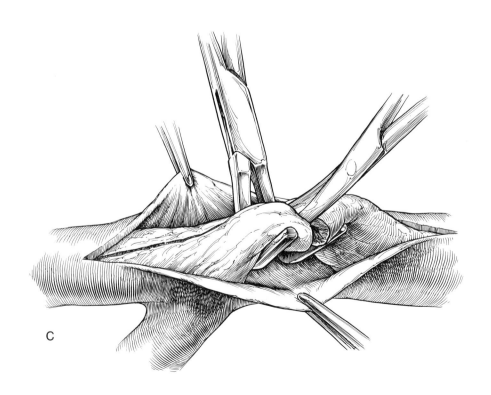

C

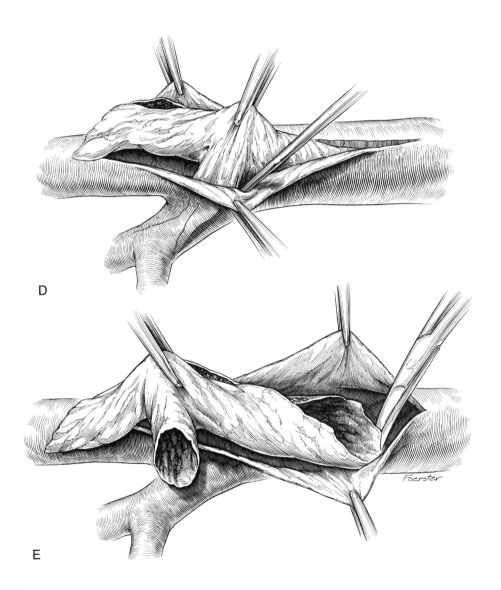

D

E

Figure 58

Typical open endarterectomy showing (A)
beginning development of correct cleavage
plane, (B) circumferentially freeing up the
plaque, (C) dividing it over a right-angle
clamp, (D) freeing it up distally into the
major outflow branches, and (E) trimming off
the proximal end of the plaque.

Basic Vascular Techniques

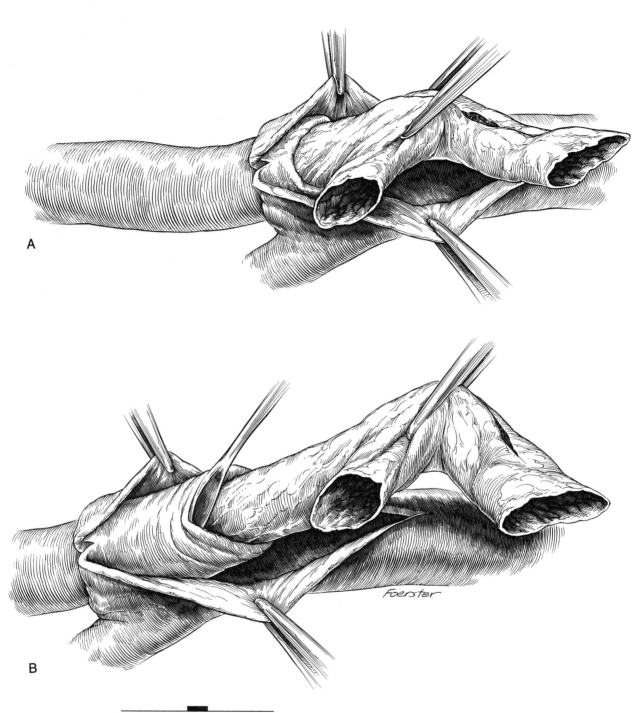

A

B

Foerster

Figure 59

Eversion endarterectomy achieved with
steady traction on the "specimen" and
opening up the correct endarterectomy
plane with the tip of the Penfield instrument
under direct vision.

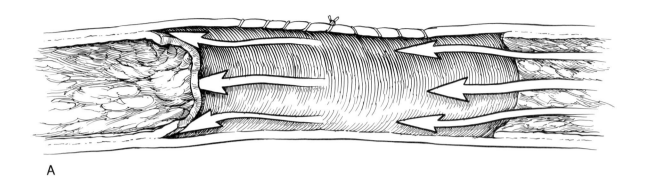

A

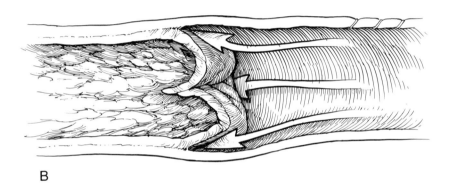

B

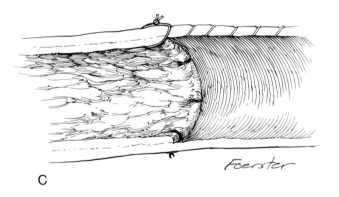

C

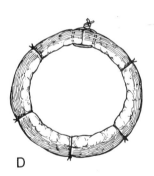

D

Foerster

Figure 60

The consequences of leaving a distal intimal "shelf." Restoring flow leads to dissection and intimal flap occlusion (A and B). Longitudinal and cross-sectional views of "tack-down" sutures to prevent this (C and D).

Basic Vascular Techniques

In instances where the disease extends for some distance down the distal vessel, the semiclosed method can be employed, using a Cannon ringed arterial stripper (Fig. 61). After the specimen has first been developed by proximal transection and trimmed of any bulky branch extensions of plaque (Fig. 61*A*), an appropriately sized Cannon ringed arterial stripper is passed over the end of the specimen and advanced downward, using a gentle, slow rotatory motion as forward pressure is applied to advance it along the natural separation plane (Fig. 61*B*). Ultimately, the stripper should suddenly "give" as it breaks into the distal lumen beyond the natural end point. The plaque should be extracted, and the distal tip of the latter inspected for satisfactory evidence that a thinly tapered end point was achieved. Additional confirmation should be sought by angioscopy or completion arteriography.

Unfortunately, the disease may extend well down the artery, even to the next convenient level of exposure. There are two options here. The first is to expose the artery distally at or just beyond the end of the major involvement and directly supervise the termination of the endarterectomy through an arteriotomy placed at that point. If the artery is still palpably thickened by atheromatous involvement, it can be obliquely transected. The endarterectomy is completed to the point of transection and the vessel reanastomosed, carefully placing the sutures from inside out all along the distal edge to tack down the intima. This approach may be used to manage superficial femoral occlusive disease if preliminary maneuvers indicate the endarterectomy plane separates easily. Rarely, it may be applied between the upper and lower popliteal artery to avoid crossing the knee with a prosthesis.

A second option is to withdraw the transected artery out through the proximal site and perform an eversion endarterectomy through its length under direct vision. Then, after cleaning off any residual fibers of media, the artery is turned back, outside-in, and the end withdrawn down to the distal site for reanastomosis. This technique has been used to advantage on the external iliac artery.

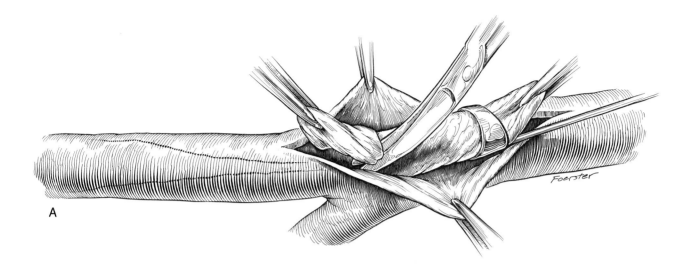

A

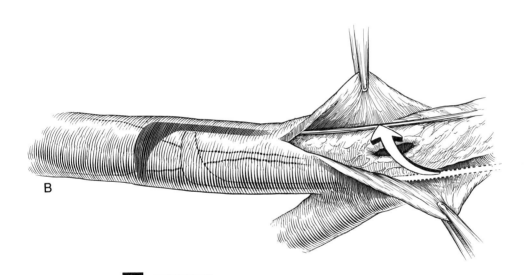

B

Figure 61

Semiclosed endarterectomy using a Cannon
ring stripper after trimming a branch from
the specimen. A gentle rotary motion is
used to assist downward insertion until the
natural end point is passed.

Basic Vascular Techniques

Finally, one may also need to manage significant orificial narrowing of a major branch when the mural disease along the adjacent wall of the main artery (e.g., aorta) is not sufficiently advanced to warrant formal endarterectomy itself. As shown in Figure 62, after the artery across from the branch orifice has been opened, the inner layer of artery can be incised to the correct depth, completely around the circumference of the opening but at a distance 2 to 3 mm wider than its lumen (Fig. 62*B*). The endarterectomy plane can then be developed with a Penfield dissector, applying traction on the specimen of stenosing plaque, as previously described, until a satisfactory end point is reached (Fig. 62*C*) and the specimen is removed (Fig. 62*D*).

On all endarterectomized surfaces, to the limit exposure permits, strips of fibers of unevenly removed outer media should be debrided before closure. They are thrombogenic and may stimulate a proliferative cellular reaction that, if excessive, progresses to myointimal hyperplasia. The fibers are transversely oriented and better stripped off in that direction, using forceps or the sweep of a peanut-sized gauze pledget grasped in the tip of a clamp.

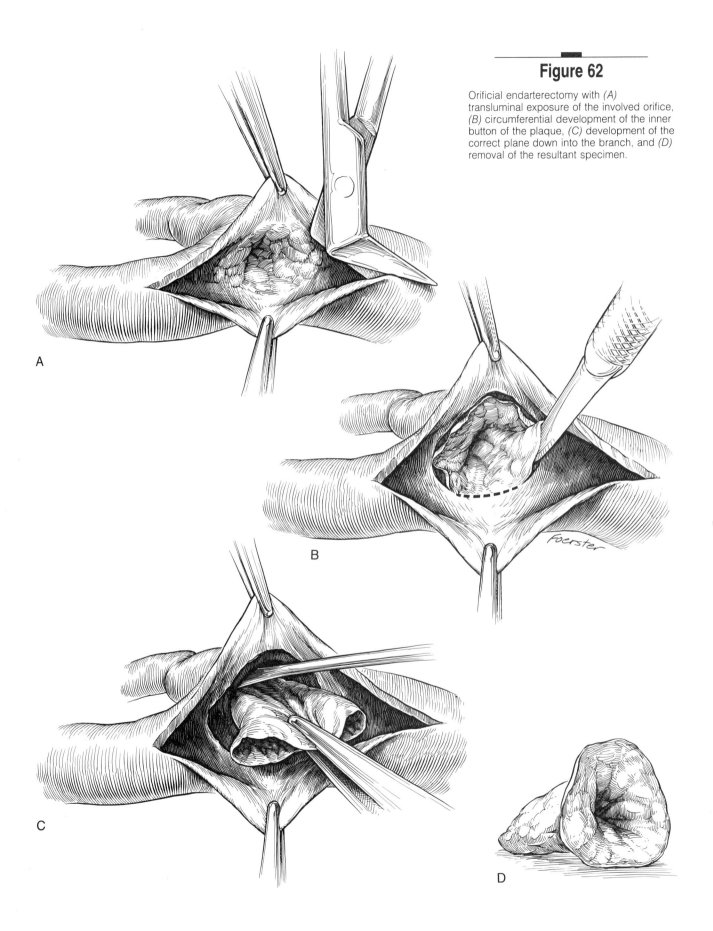

Figure 62

Orificial endarterectomy with (A) transluminal exposure of the involved orifice, (B) circumferential development of the inner button of the plaque, (C) development of the correct plane down into the branch, and (D) removal of the resultant specimen.

Basic Vascular Techniques

INTRAOPERATIVE ARTERIOGRAPHY

Determining the technical adequacy of any reconstructive or disobliterative procedure is an important, even essential, adjunctive procedure. Occasionally, it is not done with simpler procedures when the distal vessel is well exposed and can be felt to have full pulsatile flow without a thrill. Exceptions to this rule must be justified, for routine completion arteriography has revealed *unsuspected* technical flaws in up to 10 percent of arterial repairs and reconstructions. Other monitoring methods (e.g., a Doppler probe and duplex scanner) will suffice in certain situations—that is, local procedures with good exposure—but they do not detect emboli or distal obstructive lesions. Angioscopy will do this up to a point, and has other advantages, but it may be limited by caliber and lack of a proper guidance system from entering all the distal vessels. Therefore, intraoperative arteriography remains the "gold standard." How and when to do it deserves some comment. Four approaches are offered.

1. After performing an embolectomy, it is desirable to check for residual distal thrombus *before* closing the arteriotomy to avoid the necessity of reopening it should further thromboembolectomy be required. Therefore, a catheter is placed into the distal vessel and secured by "snugging up" a doubly looped Silastic tape or Rumel tourniquet (Fig. 63*A*). The amount of contrast media and the delay after injection before x-ray exposure vary. For a relatively open distal bed, the film may be exposed at the completion of a slow injection of 15 to 30 ml of full-strength (e.g., 60 percent Renografin) contrast media over 5 to 10 seconds. Timing is not as critical here because *inflow* occlusion, a common feature of intraoperative arteriography, prevents the contrast media from being rapidly flushed through the distal tree. The arteriotomy is closed after the film demonstrates an open distal arterial tree. If the arteriotomy is already closed, a simple cannula and purse-string suture are used, again with inflow occlusion (Fig. 63*B*).

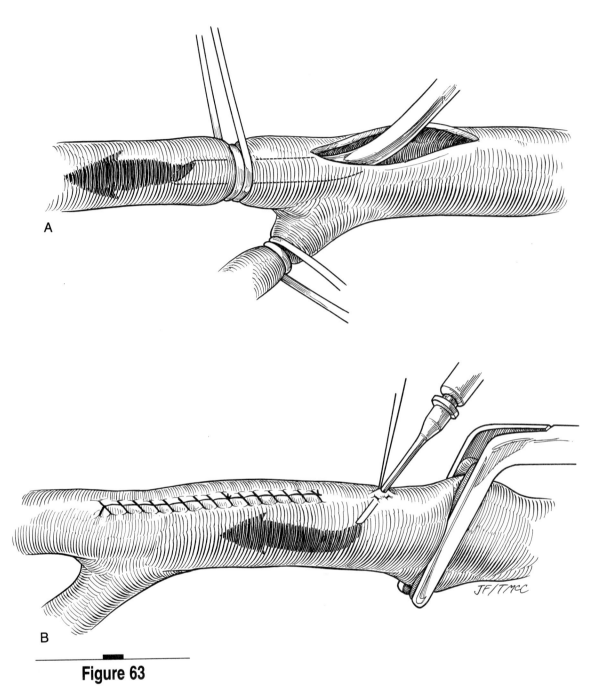

Figure 63

A, Completion arteriography after
thromboembolectomy and before
arteriotomy closure. B, Completion
arteriography after arteriotomy closure.

Basic Vascular Techniques

2. When completing a peripheral bypass, one may wish to perform arteriography *before* the final, proximal anastomosis has been performed. Problems at or near the distal anastomosis (Fig. 64*B*) or twisting or other forms of entrapment of the graft in the connecting tunnel are best dealt with at that point. Most proximal (femoral) anastomoses are easily and confidently completed under direct vision. Often, the irrigating cannula is still attached to a reversed vein graft, and this can be used to obtain arteriography of the reconstruction from this point distally, as shown in Figure 64*A*.

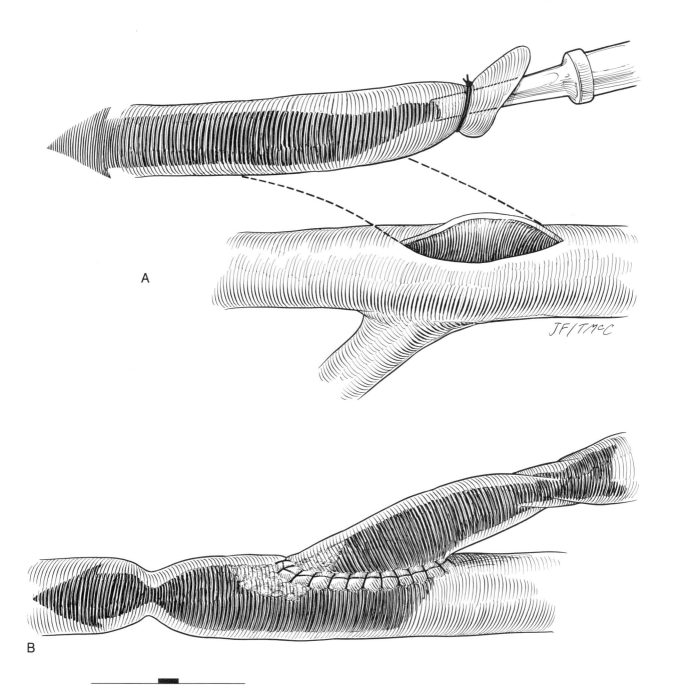

Figure 64

A, Completion arteriography after completing distal anastomosis *and* tunneling but before proximal anastomosis, via the same irrigation catheter used to dilate and test the vein graft. *B,* Demonstration of potential distal problems visualized, including twisted graft, buildup of mural thrombus at the distal anastomosis, and stricture from controlling clamp or vessel loop.

Basic Vascular Techniques

3. If one is confident enough of the reconstructive procedure or bypass, one can wait until the proximal anastomosis is almost complete and use a soft plastic catheter through the anastomotic line to obtain completion angiography (Fig. 65A).

4. Sometimes, after completing all the anastomoses, and in the case of in situ bypass after Doppler detection and closure of obvious high-flow arteriovenous communications, completion arteriography is performed as a final check before wound closure. It may be performed at this time also because Doppler evaluation of the flow through the graft and distal anastomosis, and/or over the distal (pedal) arteries, indicates that something is amiss. In this situation, one should reapply the proximal clamp, inject the contrast material through a needle or cannula inserted at the site of a proximally placed purse-string suture, and inject contrast material after occluding any side branches such as the profunda femoris with drawn-up vessel loops to direct all the contrast material through the bypass into the distal bed (Fig. 65B).

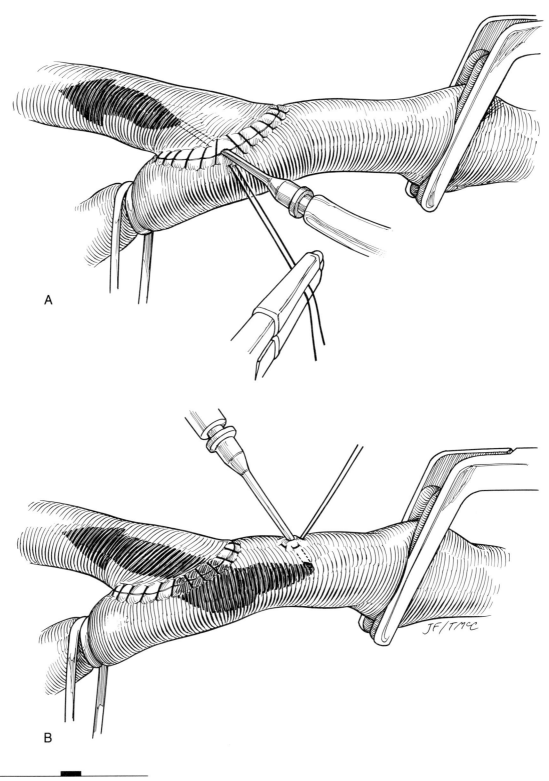

Figure 65

Intraoperative arteriography after completing
proximal anastomosis *(A)* before and *(B)*
after tying anastomotic suture.

Basic Vascular Techniques

In each of the aforementioned techniques, the following practical suggestions apply, as illustrated in Figure 66:

1. Drape the leg out so that a long narrow x-ray film cassette inside a sterile plastic cover can be easily placed under it.
2. Tether the foot in midposition for the best anteroposterior view.
3. Remove all clamps, retractors, and other metal objects from the field.
4. Use full-strength contrast media with these small volumes.
5. Stand behind an intravenous infusion pole, over which a lead apron is draped and covered with a sterile plastic bag.
6. Use extension tubing and a three-way stopcock to allow the hands to be kept away from the x-ray field and flush out the contrast media with an equal volume of heparinized saline immediately after the film is exposed.

These techniques were deliberately varied to suit the circumstances and, of course, can be varied in additional ways, but these approaches have been found to be the most useful modifications. They each feature inflow occlusion and the slow direct injection of small amounts of contrast media into relatively static distal beds, while obtaining excellent single-exposure visualization of the runoff vessels. One can take advantage of these same principles in performing intraoperative arteriography *before* beginning reconstruction, in cases of trauma or acute ischemia in which time constraints do not permit the luxury of formal preoperative arteriography in the angiography suite, or in an attempt to obtain better visualization of distal runoff vessels than achieved by preoperative arteriography. Here, a greater delay (e.g., 3 to 8 seconds) after injection may be needed before the single exposure, unless a C-arm fluoroscopy unit is available with freeze-frame feature. One should take advantage of this capability in *any* of the previous settings, when it is available.

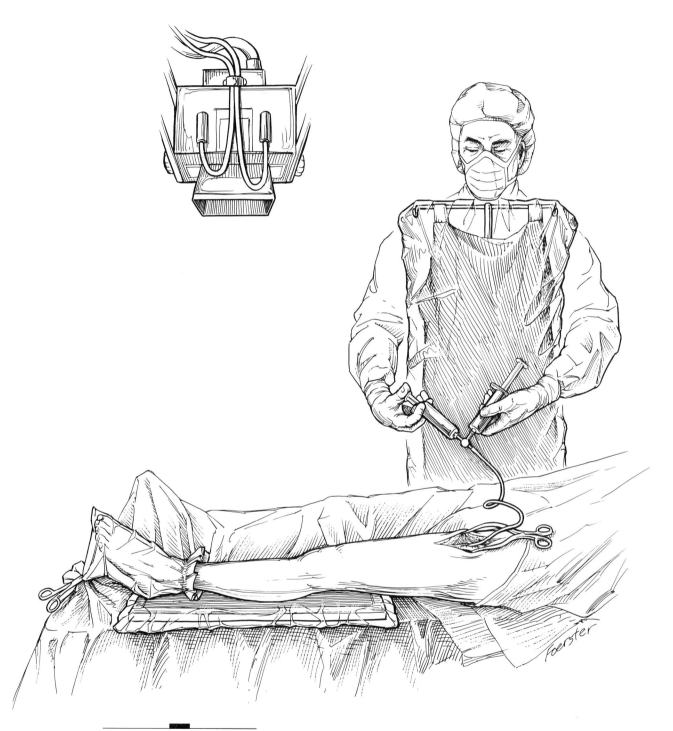

Figure 66

The major features of intraoperative
arteriography are demonstrated, including
draping and exposure of the leg, placement
of the x-ray cassette, positioning of the
overhead cathode tube, positioning of the
operator behind a sterile lead apron shield,
and extension tubing to keep the operator's
hands away from the field of exposure.

VASCULAR EXPOSURES

Vascular Exposures

This atlas began as a primer on basic vascular surgical techniques (Section 1). This section on exposures was added because exposures form the other pillar of basic technique. That is, knowing "how to get there" and "what to do when you get there" are the essential components of any surgical operation. In a temporal sense, exposure comes first, and some thought was given even to changing the order of presentation to reflect this. The other aspect of this section on exposures that received considerable thought was what was the best, most logical anatomic sequence of presenting the different exposures. Work naturally began with the most common exposure employed by vascular surgeons, the femoral vessels, and then proceeded distally in the lower extremity. One could have equally well elected to begin with a more central location, such as the infrarenal abdominal aorta. Because no sequence was clearly more logical or natural than the other, it was decided to stay with the original focus on lower extremity infrainguinal exposures, then turn to the abdominal aorta and its branches before moving upward.

There are a number of basic differences between peripheral and central exposures. The former requires a good knowledge of topographic anatomy to place the incision precisely, and then how best to move into the depths of the wound, between specific muscles, retracting them to reach the underlying neurovascular structures. For that reason, most of the illustrations of peripheral exposures begin with a topographic view with the important underlying anatomy "ghosted" in, to indicate proper incision placement. This is followed by a cross-sectional view of the anatomic pathway into the vessels before displaying stepwise exposure of the particular arterial segment of interest. Exposure of the aorta and its major branches can be carried out through a few basic incisions, the choice between which may be made on the basis of the associated pathology, the possible need for extended exposure, or simply individual preference. Unlike extremity incisions, which are potentially extensile, abdominal, flank, or thoracic incisions are deliberately extensive to begin with, the additional incision length providing an ease of exposure and operation that more than compensates for the extra minutes required for closure. Thus, the incision and muscle division stages of truncal operations are uncomplicated and much of the skill in gaining exposure for these transcavitary procedures involves mobilizing and retracting the overlying viscera, which are bulkier but more yielding than muscle. In all exposures, one must be conscious of avoiding injury to adjacent structures and choose the path with the least overlying tissues. In the periphery, adjacent nerves are a potential hazard. Centrally, adjacent viscera or their excretory conduits and blood supply may stand in the way. Finally, although historical aspects have been largely ignored, the exposures depicted here have obviously been developed by pioneers in vascular surgery to whom we all owe a great deal.

Although the choice of exposures selected for presentation in this section is the author's, no originality is claimed. Often it is difficult to remember where, or from whom, a particular approach was first acquired, but a few notable exceptions are acknowledged. It is hoped that this selection of exposures will serve the reader as well as they have the author.

EXPOSURE OF LOWER EXTREMITY VESSELS

In spite of the frequency of operations on the aorta and its major branches, and on the carotid artery and other brachiocephalic vessels, operations involving lower extremity vessels are by far the most frequent and could be called the "backbone" of vascular surgery. Exposure is usually made using extensile linear incisions, which are mostly placed over arterial segments where they are reasonably accessible and, to take advantage of the bypass principle, likely to be relatively free of occlusive disease. The incisions used to expose infrainguinal arteries that are described in the text are shown in Figure 67, which presents anterior and posterior views of the thigh, and in Figure 68, which presents infragenicular incisions used to expose the popliteal, crural, and pedal arteries.

Most bypasses performed for lower extremity ischemia begin or end at the femoral artery (e.g., aortobifemoral, axillofemoral, femorofemoral, femoropopliteal, and femorotibial bypasses). This, plus its use for embolectomy, endarterectomy, and profundaplasty, makes femoral exposure easily the most frequently utilized incision in vascular surgery. Furthermore, unless one's practice features much limb salvage and reoperative surgery, one may get by, in the majority of lower extremity revascularizations, with just three exposures: the anterior approach to the femoral arteries and the medial above- and below-knee approaches to the popliteal artery. But the complete vascular surgeon must know alternative approaches not only to these three arterial segments but also to the tibial vessels at all levels, and even beyond, to the pedal arteries.

In some cases dissection can be guided by frequent referral to an underlying arterial pulse, but in most cases associated arterial occlusive disease precludes using this clue. Therefore, one needs other, more reliable anatomic landmarks for the incision. In addition, choosing the easiest pathway into the underlying vessels requires a practical knowledge of regional anatomy, particularly the relative positions of each of the neurovascular triad, the artery, vein, and nerve, and their relationships to nearby muscles. For this reason, most of the exposures illustrated in this part of the atlas each feature (1) the relationships of the incision to topographic landmarks and underlying anatomy and (2) the cross-sectional view of the anatomy at the level of the incision, showing the relationship between the neurovascular structures and adjacent muscles, as well as the correct anatomic route between incision and vessels. Then the major steps of exposure are depicted, ending with full isolation and control, using loops or tapes, of the main vessel itself. For uniformity, only *right*-sided extremity exposures are illustrated.

Some general advice given in Section 1 regarding exposure of extremity vessels is offered again here:

1. Make incisions of adequate length.
2. Use self-retaining retractors with adequate depth and grasp, and readjust them at each level of exposure.
3. Beware of nerve injury, not only from cutting instruments but also from poorly placed clamps, retractors, and particularly nearby use of cautery (when the current is left at the usual level employed in abdominal or chest exposures).
4. Be aware of the lymphatics, coursing close to the veins and arteries, and, if they are to be transected, ligate or cauterize the divided ends.
5. Even pulseless arteries can be located in surrounding fat or scar tissue, either by palpation (a firm tubular structure if occluded) or by Doppler localization (if patent beyond an occlusion).
6. As soon as feasible, dissect close to and then around the artery. Then traction on an encircling umbilical tape will bring the artery up into the field and allow other, extraneous structures to be more readily dissected away. This is much safer than trying to fully dissect out a vessel lying in its bed in the depths of the wound.

Vascular Exposures

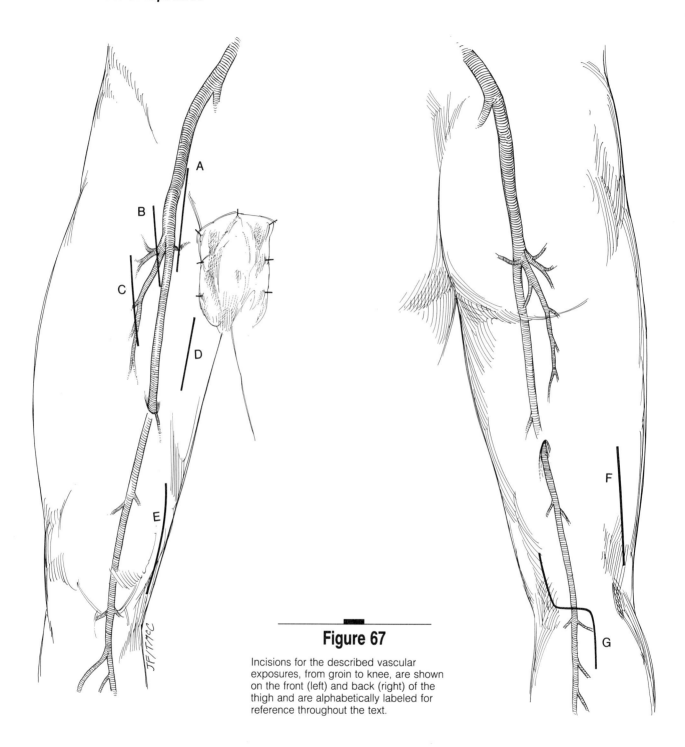

Figure 67

Incisions for the described vascular
exposures, from groin to knee, are shown
on the front (left) and back (right) of the
thigh and are alphabetically labeled for
reference throughout the text.

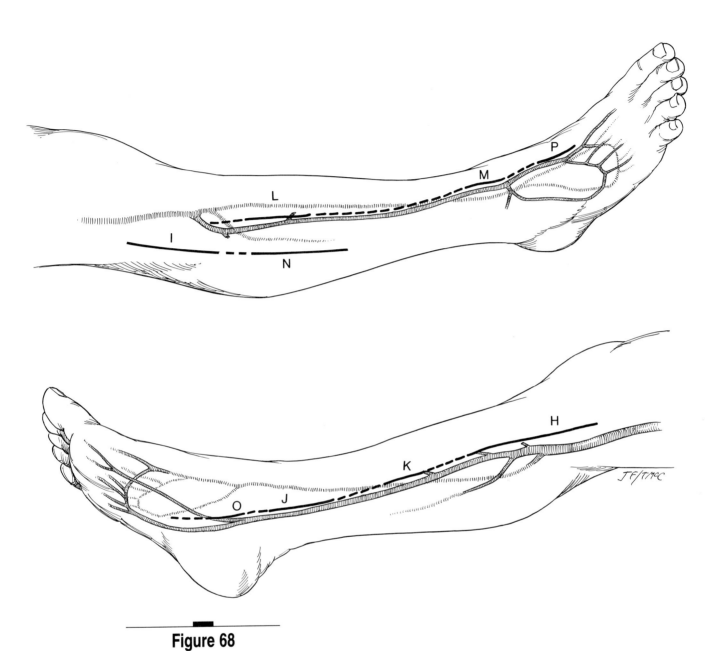

Figure 68

Incisions for infragenicular vascular
exposures are shown in anterolateral
(above) and posteromedial (below) views of
the lower leg. Alphabetic labels refer to
sequential discussion in the text.

Vascular Exposures

Infrainguinal Exposures

Exposure of the Femoral Vessels (Incision A; Fig. 67). The most commonly used femoral groin incision is shown on the left side of Figure 69*A*. On the right side of Figure 69*A* are several alternatives, one of which is an oblique incision, 1 cm below and parallel to the inguinal crease. This incision may be more cosmetically acceptable, and it serves adequately if only a limited exposure of the femoral bifurcation is needed, but it requires more extensive division of lymphatics and therefore carries a higher risk of lymphedema, lymphocele, or lymph fistula. To avoid these complications, one may dissect in vertical planes once the superficial fascia has been opened but, again, the exposure is quite limited.

Another oblique incision, for use only in the very obese, is shown in Figure 69*B*. Vertical incisions in such patients, particularly those with diabetes, are often plagued by superficial wound infection and the intertriginous area may become macerated and difficult to manage. By making an oblique incision *on top of the panniculus* but still directly overlying the femoral vessels, one can approach them from above (as shown in a side view in Figure 69*C*) and avoid these annoying groin wound problems. Using downward traction on the lower panniculus, the lower fibers of the external oblique aponeurosis are identified and followed down to the inguinal ligament and beyond, to the common femoral artery. Through this incision the *proximal* superficial and deep femoral arteries can be reached and controlled, but they represent the distal limits of this exposure.

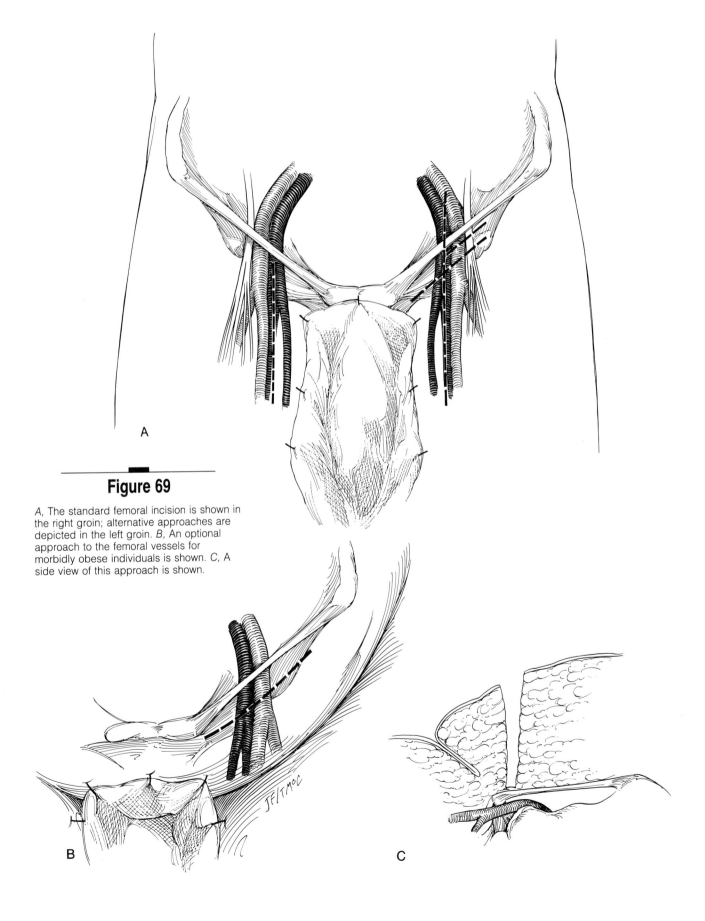

Figure 69

A, The standard femoral incision is shown in the right groin; alternative approaches are depicted in the left groin. *B,* An optional approach to the femoral vessels for morbidly obese individuals is shown. *C,* A side view of this approach is shown.

Vascular Exposures

However, in the majority of circumstances, the standard vertical femoral incision is made. The commonly used landmark for this is the pubic tubercle, with the femoral artery lying approximately 2 fingerbreaths (FB) lateral to this (Fig. 70*A*). If only limited exposure is needed, as for a femoral embolectomy, the incision can begin at the inguinal crease and be carried 4 to 5 FB distally, inclining slightly medially, aimed at the medial aspect of the knee. However, to gain full exposure of the common femoral vessels, this incision should be carried *well above the inguinal crease* (which lies lower than the inguinal ligament), exposing and, if necessary, cutting the lowermost fibers of the external oblique aponeurosis. For this additional upward exposure, the skin incision may be extended straight upward, vertically, or angled off laterally, parallel to the inguinal crease, as shown on the right side of Figure 69*A*. Distal external iliac exposure requires cutting additional fibers of the external oblique aponeurosis and retracting the underlying muscle and peritoneal sac upward and medially. Additional distal extension of the skin incision may be required for femoral profundaplasty.

Although the femoral artery is often pulseless when the intended procedure is being performed for proximal occlusive disease (e.g., aortobifemoral or femorofemoral bypass) or for an embolus, it can usually be felt, even through the skin, as a firm tubular structure when rolled under the fingers, as shown in Figure 70*B* and *C*, because of firm clot and/or atheromatous plaque. The artery lies just lateral to the bottom of the trough formed by the iliopsoas and pectineus muscles.

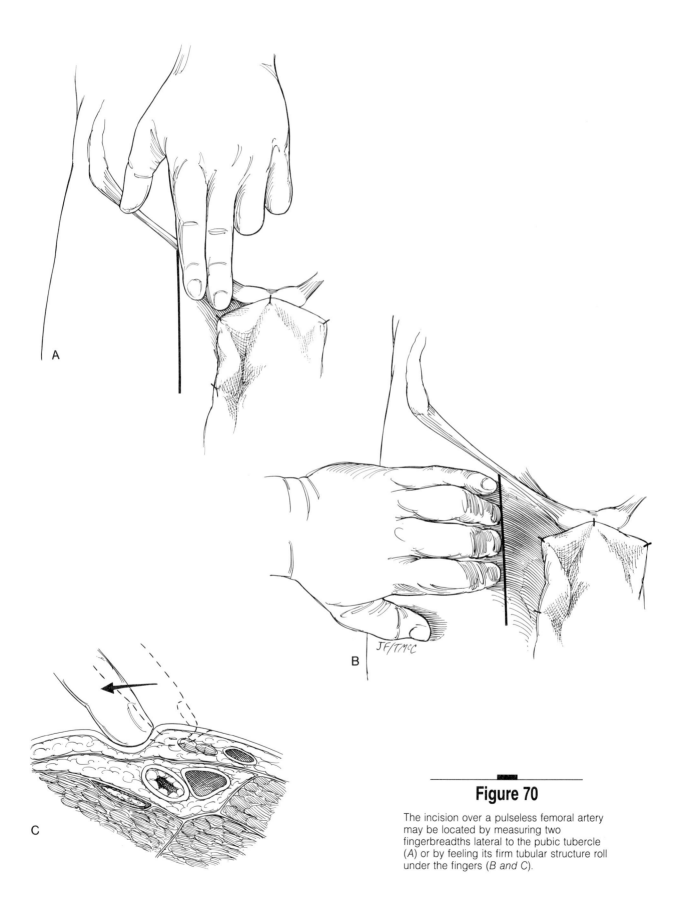

Figure 70

The incision over a pulseless femoral artery may be located by measuring two fingerbreadths lateral to the pubic tubercle (A) or by feeling its firm tubular structure roll under the fingers (B and C).

Vascular Exposures

After the initial skin incision is made and the superficial fascia opened, lateral tributaries of the greater saphenous vein may be encountered (Fig. 71A), and these must be ligated and divided. If exposure of the saphenous vein itself will be required for the reconstruction, one of these ligatures can be cut long, on the medial side of the largest divided branch, so that it may later serve as a marker when that part of the dissection begins. In anatomy courses, students are often taught to remember the relationships in the femoral canal by using the mnemonic NAVEL: *N*erve–*A*rtery–*V*ein–*E*mpty space–*L*ymphatics. Although this may be true of relationships deeper in the femoral canal, more superficially one will find inguinal lymph nodes and their lymphatic tributaries lying both medial and lateral to the saphenous vein. If possible one should stay lateral to these nodes in approaching the femoral artery. If the greater saphenous vein will later be used, one can then dissect medial to the lymphatics, just *under* the superficial fascia, before dissecting downward to expose this vein, thereby leaving a "bridge" of intact lymphatics inbetween (Fig. 71B). Even with these precautions some lymphatics will usually be transected, particularly as the exposure proceeds upward (more proximally). Therefore, tissues in this area should be ligated in continuity or at least divided with the cautery, using the coagulation setting.

Following the aforementioned landmarks, and carrying dissection deeper in the described vertical plane, one can expose the femoral artery by opening the vascular sheath covering it. This sheath is an extension or duplication of the deep fascia. If, upon opening what is thought to be the femoral sheath, one sees underlying muscle (the iliopsoas) or fibers of the femoral nerve, one is too far lateral. Encountering venous structures and accompanying deep lymphatics indicates one is too far medial. But straying medially or laterally should not occur if one frequently feels for the pulse or, in its absence, either rolls the firm occluded artery under the fingers or uses a hand-held Doppler to locate the artery, patent beyond a proximal occlusion. If there is no Doppler arterial signal, spontaneous sounds from the femoral *vein,* which lies directly medial to it, can be used for orientation. These measures should allow the artery to be readily exposed even under difficult circumstances. Similar techniques can be applied to all extremity vascular exposures if one knows the basic anatomic relationships and uses frequent palpation or Doppler soundings.

After the overlying fascial sheath is opened, the exposed artery will be quickly recognized by the unique pattern of the vasa vasorum on its surface, a mosaic that only a peripheral artery possesses. Whether the segment first encountered is the superficial or the common femoral artery may be readily apparent from its caliber and one's proximity to the upper or lower end of the incision. If not, after encircling the artery with an umbilical tape and using traction on this, dissection should be carried proximally. When one encounters an abrupt change in caliber, this marks the femoral bifurcation and locates the origin of the profunda femoris, which is usually not readily visible at first because it courses posteriorly and slightly laterally from this point. Distal to the bifurcation, a sensory branch of the femoral nerve may cross the superficial femoral artery from lateral to medial. It should be protected to avoid medial thigh discomfort postoperatively (Fig. 71C).

To obtain control of all three components of the femoral bifurcation, it is best to encircle the common and superficial femoral arteries first, then to use upward traction on the surrounding tapes to draw the profunda femoris up from its bed. If it is still difficult to pass a right-angle clamp completely around it, the profunda can be more safely encircled by first passing a tape under the superficial femoral below the profunda, and then passing the other end of the same tape under the common femoral above the profunda, both from medial to lateral. With traction on these two ends, the now encircled profunda femoris can be readily lifted up and, if desired, an additional loop of the same tape can be passed around it to create a Potts loop. This second loop can be performed in a similar manner, passing the upper end back medially under the superficial femoral and then laterally again under the common femoral, to complete the second encirclement. This double encirclement sequence, used to create a Potts loop around a major deep branch that lies adjacent to major veins, is illustrated later in the exposure of the iliac bifurcation, where the risk of venous injury is particularly worrisome (see Fig. 91A through F).

For more complete exposure, such as that shown in Figure 71D, one can dissect further proximally and distally from the bifurcation. The common femoral artery rarely has any deep branches other than the profunda itself, except for the occasional anomalous origin of one of the profunda branches. However, it does have one or two lateral branches higher up near the inguinal ligament, and these will be larger than normal if they have developed as collaterals in response to occlusive disease. They should be double-looped with a heavy silk suture.

The superficial femoral artery is usually easily freed up, having only occasional small "twigs" in its upper portion, but the profunda femoris cannot be so readily freed up, first because of its lateral circumflex iliac branch, which usually leaves it just beyond its origin, and second because of the lateral circumflex iliac vein which, after leaving the femoral vein and coursing under the superficial femoral artery, crosses *on top of* the profunda femoris artery less than an inch down from its origin. This vein may not be readily seen and may be inadvertently incised, because upward traction on the tape surrounding the profunda femoris artery will compress and empty this vein, so that the usual warning blueness, seen when approaching a vein, is absent. It should be specifically sought, identified, and divided. This maneuver will allow full exposure of the first part of the profunda femoris and somewhat beyond, down to the upper muscular and perforating branches (Fig. 71D, E).

Vascular Exposures

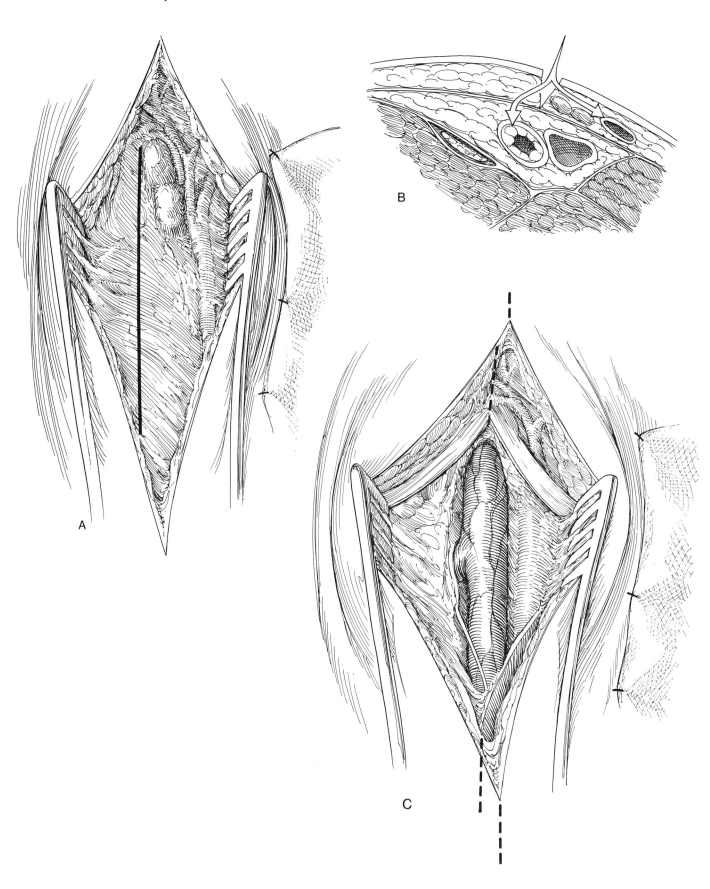

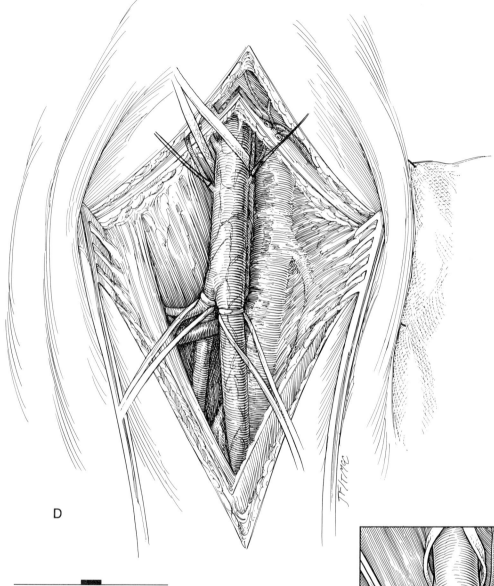

D

Figure 71

A, With the skin and superficial fascia incised, the dissection plane should be deepened lateral to the saphenous vein and inguinal nodes (solid line). B, If the saphenous vein also requires exposure, a route *medial* to the nodes is chosen, leaving an intact bridge of lymphatic tissue between it and the femoral artery, which lies deeper within a sheath of investing deep fascia. C, Deeper exposure of the femoral bifurcation may require longitudinal extensions of the superficial layers, especially in obese individuals. A branch of the femoral nerve may occasionally cross the upper superficial femoral artery anteriorly and should be avoided. D, Final exposure of the femoral bifurcations shows the proximity of the femoral vein medially, two to four small arterial branches medially and laterally as the inguinal ligament is approached and incised, and the lateral circumflex iliac vein crossing over the first part of the profunda femoris artery. Prior to opening the common femoral artery, its branches are double-looped with Silastic tapes or, if small, with heavy silk ligatures, and an umbilical tape is placed proximally for traction while applying a vascular clamp. E, If exposure of the proximal profunda femoris artery is also required, as for profundaplasty, the overlying vein must be divided between ligatures and small Silastic loops are placed on the appropriate profunda artery branches.

Vascular Exposures

Exposure of the Femoral Vein

Exposure of the femoral vein utilizes a similar vertical skin and superficial fascia incision to that utilized to expose the artery, but one first identifies the saphenous vein and follows it down to the femoral vein. Therefore, the skin incision should be placed more medially, by about 1 FB, because the most reliable landmark for the saphenofemoral junction is a point 1 inch lateral and 1 inch distal from the pubic tubercle (Fig. 72*A*). Ordinarily, one should stay on the *lateral* side of the saphenous vein as one dissects downward, preserving it to one side. The upper part of the dissection is similar to that used for high ligation or "harvest" of the greater saphenous vein, but as one proceeds deeper and enters the fossa ovalis, incising its lower rim to expose the underlying femoral vein, the superficial external pudendal artery traverses this rim and must be ligated before division (Fig. 72*B*). Otherwise, the overlying tissues can be divided proximally and distally with relative impunity to expose the femoral vein. One will find the superficial and deep femoral veins, each with a sentinel valve, joining to form the common femoral vein an inch or two below the saphenofemoral junction, but there are often one to three sizable tributaries entering near the bifurcation that also must be isolated and controlled (Fig. 72*C*). Obviously, traction and dissection must be gentler than when exposing the femoral artery.

Exposure of the Distal Profunda Femoris Artery (Incisions B, C, D; Fig. 67)

Increasingly, the second and third parts of the profunda femoris artery are being utilized as the origin or termination of bypass grafts, particularly in reoperative surgery, when the proximal femoral vessels are often imbedded in scar tissue or inflammatory reaction. As Frank Veith has pointed out, not only does this approach allow avoidance of the inherent difficulties of returning to the scene of lost battles nearby, but also the distal profunda femoris artery serves well as the proximal anastomotic site for a distal bypass graft when dealing with a limited length of autologous vein. For example, a full length of *lesser* saphenous vein (approximately 40 cm) usually reaches from the distal profunda to the upper tibial arteries. Typically, this segment of profunda femoris is less diseased than the proximal artery and, when the superficial femoris artery is chronically occluded, compensatory enlargement of the profunda femoris makes it quite large enough to serve as an inflow site (e.g., 4 to 5 mm in diameter).

Just as the reasons for choosing the distal profunda femoris may differ, so can the approach to accommodate these goals. However, the graft route is usually the overriding consideration. This is best appreciated by studying Figure 73*A*. For grafts entering or leaving laterally, such as an axillary-profunda or profunda-anterior tibial bypass, an anterolateral approach (B) is preferred. For a femoral-profunda crossover bypass graft, one would use an anteromedial approach (C), but if the graft is to go from the profunda down to the popliteal or the posterior tibial artery, either the anteromedial (C) or the posteromedial (D) approach could be used. However, the posteromedial approach adequately exposes only the distal third of the profunda femoris artery, so that the caliber of the distal segments of this vessel must also be considered in making this decision.

The upper two skin incisions, to expose the middle and distal thirds, can be made along either the lateral (B) or the medial (C) border of the sartorius muscle (Fig. 73*A*), proceeding around that muscle before continuing deeply into the valley between the vastus medialis and the adductor longus muscles (cross section, Fig. 73*B*). Or one can approach the third part of the profunda femoris artery medially, *behind* the adductor longus muscle, using the lower incision (D) shown in Figure 73*A*. This approach is described later.

In either the *anterolateral* or the *anteromedial* approach, after the sartorius muscle is mobilized and retracted to one side, the dissection proceeds deeply, passing lateral to the superficial femoral vessels and accompanying nerves, to the bottom of the valley between the vastus medialis (laterally) and the adductor longus muscle (medially) where a raphe, formed by the intercussating fibers from their respective fasciae, is encountered (Fig. 73*C*). Once this is opened, the profunda femoris vessels will be found directly underneath, unfortunately with the vein on top (Fig. 73*D*). It may be necessary to divide one or two venous branches to reach and isolate a segment of the artery (Fig. 73*E*).

Vascular Exposures

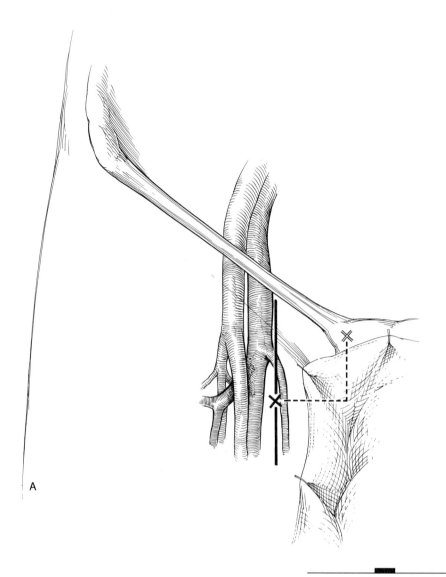

A

Figure 72

A, Femoral vein exposure is made more medially than femoral artery exposure and is keyed on the upper greater saphenous vein, located 1 inch lateral to and 1 inch below the pubic tubercle. *B,* The plane is deepened just lateral to the saphenous vein, dividing its lateral branches (dotted line). In opening through the inferior edge of the fossa ovalis (curved dotted line), the superficial external pudendal artery is usually encountered. *C,* When finally exposed and controlled with loops and tapes, the common femoral vein and its three major tributaries will be seen to have valves at their upper ends. The common femoral vein's "sentinel" valve is the upper venous valve of the lower extremity (except for an occasional iliac valve), but it may be missing in 25 to 33 percent of individuals; this will contribute to the formation of greater saphenous varicosities.

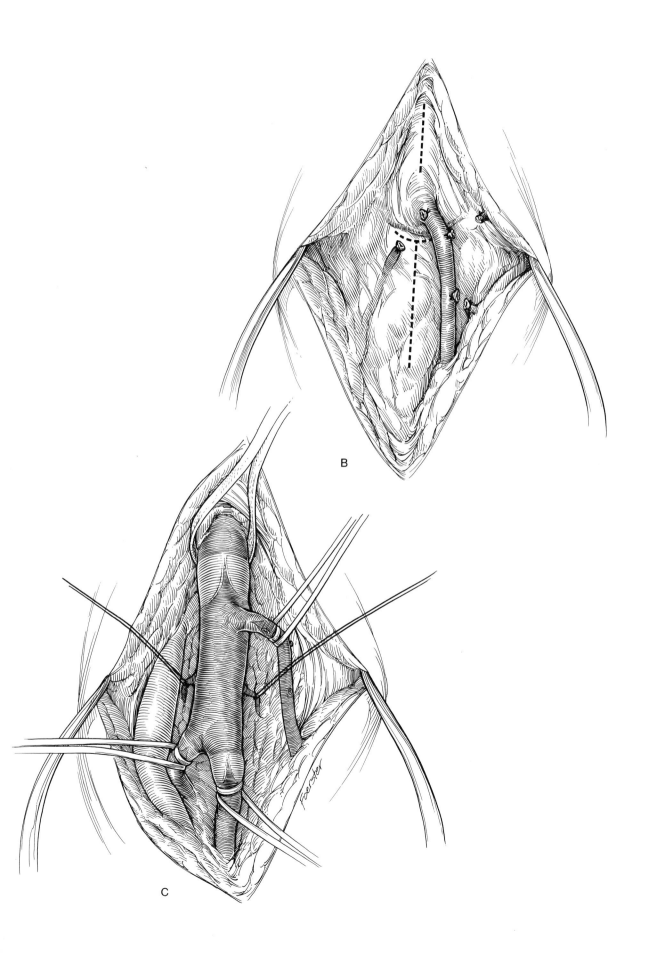

B

C

Vascular Exposures

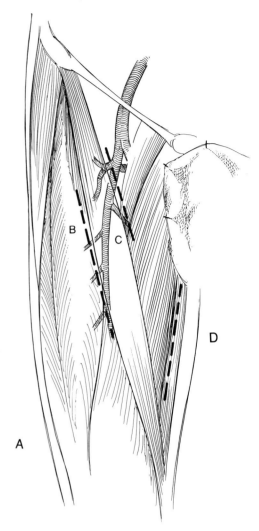

A

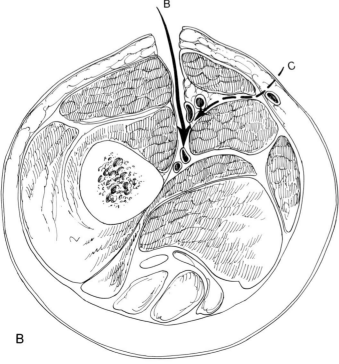

B

Figure 73

A, Three different incisions (marked B, C, and D, according to Figure 67) are shown, which can be used to expose the middle and/or distal thirds of the profunda femoris artery. *B,* A cross-sectional view showing the anterolateral (B) and anteromedial (C) approaches, passing lateral and medial to the sartorius muscle, respectively, and to one side of the superficial femoral vessels, to reach the profunda femoris artery. *C,* After passing deep to the superficial femoral vessels, between the vastus medialis and the adductor longus muscles, a raphe will be found barring the way to the profunda femoris vessels. *D,* When this raphe is incised, the profunda femoris vessels will be encountered, vein uppermost. *E,* After dividing a few branches of the adjacent vein, the profunda femoris artery can be exposed and controlled with encircling tapes.

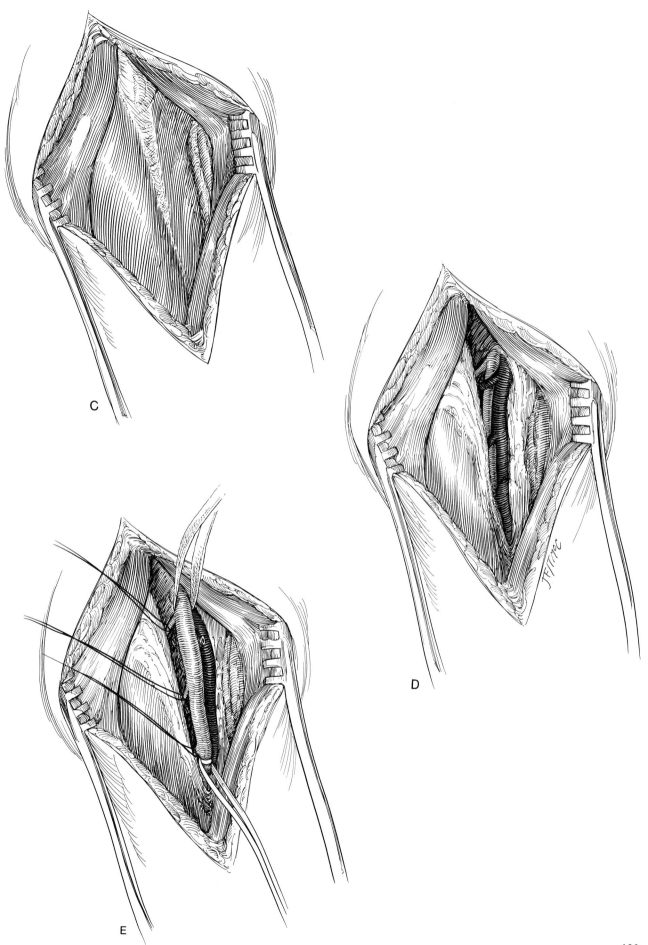

C

D

E

129

Vascular Exposures

The *posteromedial* approach (incision D in Figs. 67 and 73*A*) is made through an incision spanning the second fifth of a line from the upper groin to the medial aspect of the knee (Fig. 74*A*). For this approach, the pelvis should be slightly tilted (opposite side up) and the thigh externally rotated, with the knee flexed. By dissecting posterior to the adductor longus muscle and following the route shown in Figure 74*B*, the deep femoral vessels will be encountered near the inner (lateral) margin of that muscle, with the vein placed superiorly (Fig. 74*C*), allowing easier access to the artery than with the previously described anterior approaches. This approach is actually not significantly deeper than the anterior approaches and, with the knee flexed and the muscles relaxed, it gives ready access (Fig. 74*D*). The main disadvantages are that the approach exposes only the distal third of the profunda femoris and allows only medial entry.

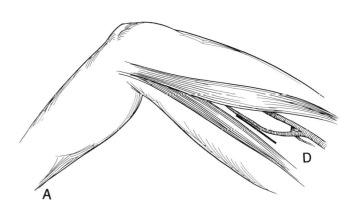

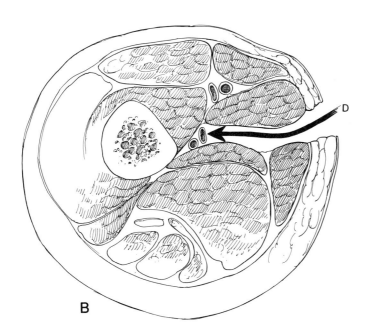

Figure 74

A, The incision for posteromedial exposure of the distal profunda femoris artery (D) is placed along the second fifth of a line from the pubic tubercle to the medial femoral condyle. *B*, A cross-sectional view showing the proper route for this incision (D, in Fig. 67), traveling immediately beneath the lower aspect of the adductor longus muscle. *C*, Exposure of distal profunda femoris and vein through this approach. *D*, Mobilization and control are made easier because the accompanying vein is out of the way, above the artery.

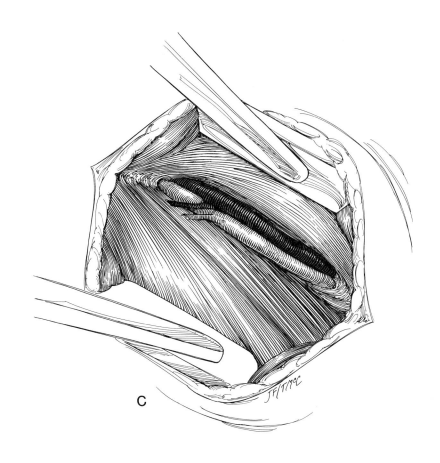

C

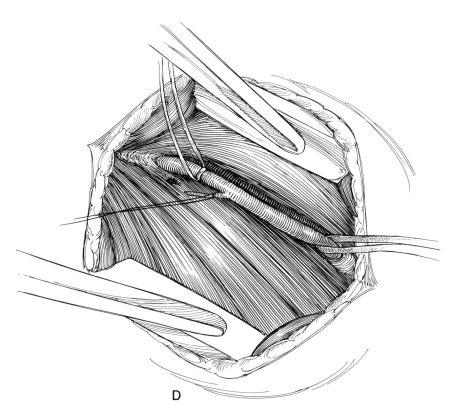

D

Vascular Exposures

Medial Exposure of the Above-Knee Popliteal Artery (Incision E; Fig. 67)

This exposure is most commonly used for femoropopliteal bypass terminating above the knee. The level of the incision is best located by palpating the lower edge of the vastus medialis, as shown in Figure 75A (solid line). If one intends to use the greater saphenous vein as the bypass graft, it is better to place the incision a little more posteriorly (dotted line), half the distance between the first location (solid line) and the course of the greater saphenous vein, which can be marked on the skin if ultrasound mapping is performed preoperatively.

When the incision is deepened, one will encounter the deep fascia near the point of attachment of the medial intermuscular septum (Fig. 75B). The fascia should be opened *below* this level to gain direct access to the popliteal fossa; otherwise, one will have to also open the intermuscular septum to reach the popliteal vessels. As one creates and enlarges this opening, it must be remembered that the saphenous nerve is likely to be encountered here, for, just after it emerges with the popliteal vessels through the hiatus in the tendon of the adductor magnus muscle, it passes steadily outward to join the saphenous vein near the knee. It is usually found near the small vessels that cross this space proximally as one approaches the adductor canal and, if they are inadvertently cut, the nerve can be caught and crushed when clamping their bleeding ends. It can also be inadvertently divided at the distal end of the incision if it courses above the fascial incision and the latter is then blindly extended distally. If one adds to the foregoing, cautery injury and entrapment during fascial closure, there are several ways of injuring the saphenous nerve and, unless these are kept in mind, there may be a significant number of postoperative complaints related to this incision. The anesthetic area produced by complete nerve division is annoying, but the causalgic pain produced by partial injury, or the shooting pains of entrapment, are intolerable.

A finger can be inserted into the popliteal space through this fascial opening between the vastus medialis and the sartorius muscles and the popliteal artery palpated up against the femur even when there is no pulse, because arteriosclerotic changes or thrombus will make it firmer than the other surrounding structures (Fig. 75C). The sciatic nerve is also firm but more flat and rubbery to the touch and, of course, more deeply located. Next, it is best to select the closest, most available segment of the popliteal artery and, staying in the areolar tissue plane close to its adventitia, dissect around it and encircle it with a moistened umbilical tape, using traction to draw it up out of its bed. Then one can dissect away the surrounding tissues, and, rather than explore the entire segment deep in its bed while seeking the best area to locate an anastomosis, one can readily palpate in either direction for the most pliant segment with the artery drawn up into the wound and then quickly redirect the dissection.

Characteristically, the popliteal vessels lie in the considerable amount of adipose tissue that fills the popliteal space. Furthermore, the artery, as is increasingly true of peripheral arteries as one proceeds distally, is surrounded by a network of *closely* applied venae comitantes (Fig. 75D). By dividing one or two of these little veins between ligatures, the rest of the network will usually dissect away without further difficulty, provided the dissection stays in the periadventitial plane. Genicular artery branches should be preserved by encircling them with a double-looped heavy silk suture, to the ends of which a clamp is attached, its weight serving as adequate traction to control backbleeding. The final exposure is seen in Figure 75E.

Popliteal Vein Exposure. If the artery is mobilized up out of its bed this way, the popliteal vein is often not even seen, though it lies directly behind and slightly below the artery. If the vein is the focus of attention, its dissection is facilitated by first applying traction on the artery. The vein can then be dissected free without rough handling, using a soft Silastic loop for gentle traction (Fig. 75F).

Obtaining Additional Proximal and Distal Exposure. Exposure of the above-knee popliteal artery, from the adductor hiatus all the way down to the point of genuflexion, can usually be obtained by further bending the knee and extending the skin and fascial incision another inch or two distally. Because of angulation on an anteroposterior x-ray film, this midpopliteal point is at the midpatella level as seen on the arteriogram, not at the level of the joint space. One cannot reach much beyond this level to make an anastomosis through this incision without taking down most of the medially inserting muscles and tendons, but by bending the knee it is usually not necessary to divide fibers of the gastrocnemius muscle or violate the pes anserinus and the underlying extension of the joint synovium in order to expose the *above-knee* popliteal artery. However, additional exposure may be necessary, as in the direct medial approach to *complicated* popliteal aneurysms that cannot simply be treated by bypass plus exclusion. Many vascular surgeons, believing that all the medial muscles attaching around the knee can be separated from their origins or insertions with impunity, do not bother to reattach them. This may be true in most of the elderly patients operated upon for limb salvage, but the author prefers either to avoid dividing them or to reattach them at the time of closure, using a technique developed by orthopedists of fixating their common base back onto the bone with heavy staples.

Occasionally, it is necessary to reach the distal superficial femoral artery just *above* the adductor hiatus, as in performing a "short" femorotibial bypass, when the proximal artery is patent and reasonably disease free immediately above the adductor hiatus. To do this, the tendinous rim of the adductor tendon must be divided, after first ligating the overlying vessels and identifying and protecting the saphenous nerve.

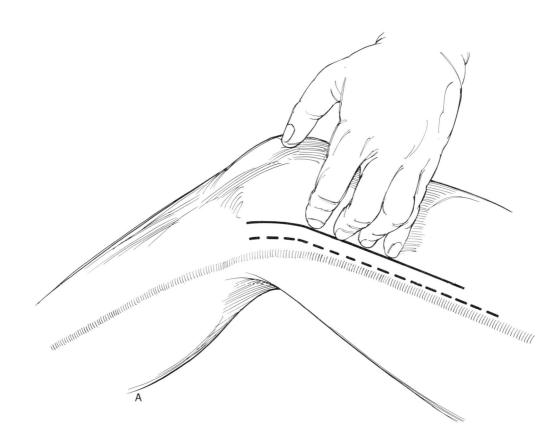

A

Figure 75

A, The medial incision to expose the popliteal artery above the knee is made longitudinally over the palpable depression between the vastus medialis above and the sartorius below (solid line). If the greater saphenous vein (shaded outline) will be needed, the incision can be made closer to it (dotted line). *B,* Once the skin and superficial fascia are opened, the deep fascia will be seen as well as the more opaque outline of its junction with the medial intermuscular septum. The fascia is incised below (posterior) to this junction, as indicated by the dotted line.

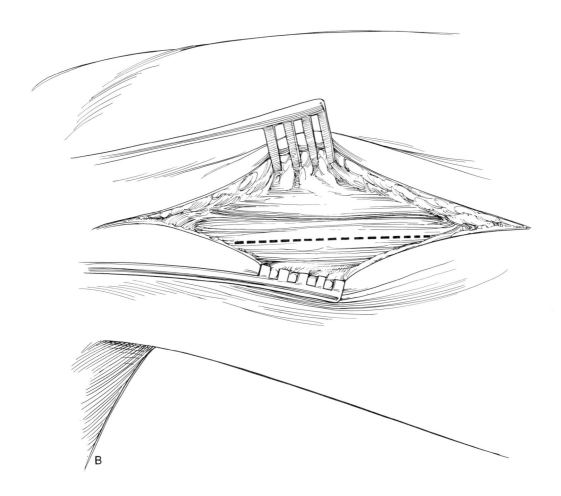

B

Vascular Exposures

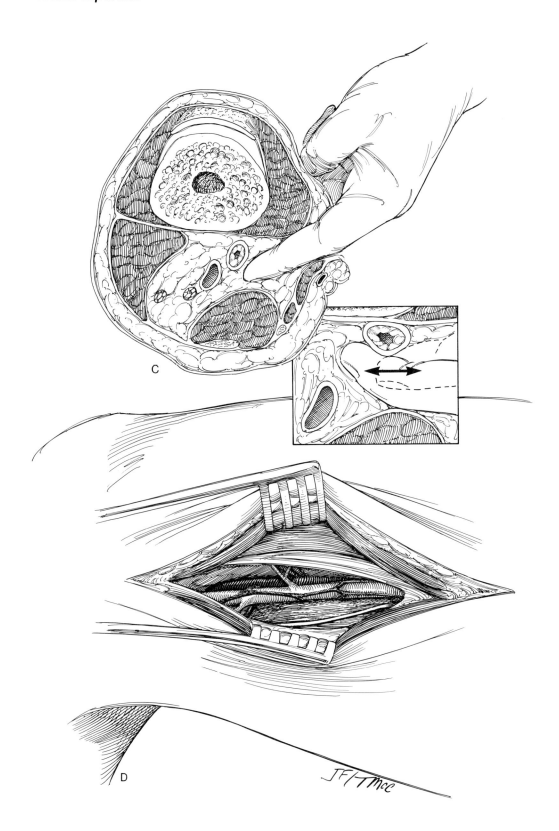

C

D

JF/TMcc

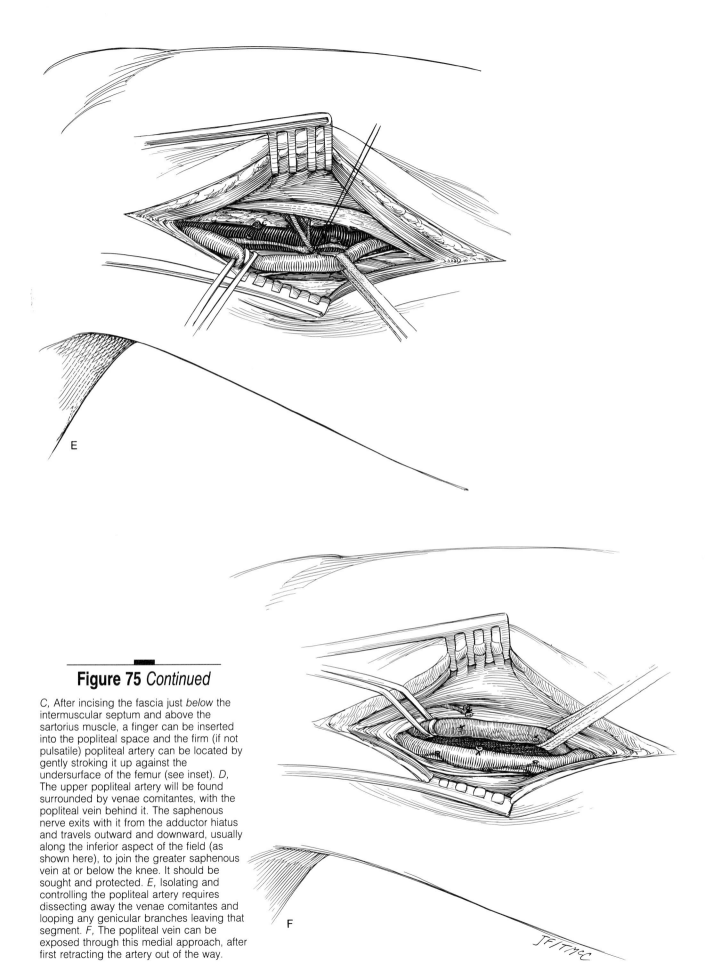

Figure 75 *Continued*

C, After incising the fascia just *below* the intermuscular septum and above the sartorius muscle, a finger can be inserted into the popliteal space and the firm (if not pulsatile) popliteal artery can be located by gently stroking it up against the undersurface of the femur (see inset). *D,* The upper popliteal artery will be found surrounded by venae comitantes, with the popliteal vein behind it. The saphenous nerve exits with it from the adductor hiatus and travels outward and downward, usually along the inferior aspect of the field (as shown here), to join the greater saphenous vein at or below the knee. It should be sought and protected. *E,* Isolating and controlling the popliteal artery requires dissecting away the venae comitantes and looping any genicular branches leaving that segment. *F,* The popliteal vein can be exposed through this medial approach, after first retracting the artery out of the way.

Vascular Exposures

Lateral Approach to the Above-Knee Popliteal Artery (Incision F; Fig. 67)

As pointed out by Frank Padberg, Jr., this approach has advantages over the usual medial approach in a limited number of special circumstances; for example, as a lateral approach for axillopopliteal bypass, chosen when the femoral area is infected or badly scarred and when all the components of the femoral bifurcation are chronically occluded, when infection or scar preclude the medial above-knee approach, and when performing the proximal anastomosis of a popliteal-to-anterior tibial or peroneal bypass, in which the use of a simple lateral subcutaneous route is obviously advantageous.

As seen in Figure 76*A*, the incision is placed longitudinally, so as to enter between the vastus lateralis and the biceps femoris muscles, for a distance of 6 to 8 FB proximal to the lateral femoral condyle. The route between these muscles enters the popliteal fossa and reaches the popliteal vessels at about the same depth as the medial approach, but here the sciatic nerve and popliteal vein will be encountered *before* reaching the popliteal artery (Fig. 76*B*). The only other unique aspect to this approach is that the dense overlying fascia lata cannot be simply incised if a graft will enter or leave by this route. It will have to be generously "T-ed" at each end of the incision (Fig. 76*C*) or partially excised to gain full exposure and avoid graft impingement. Final exposure (Fig. 76*D*) is achieved by first retracting the sciatic nerve downward and then dissecting the popliteal vein away from the popliteal artery in the same direction, dividing anterior branches, if any, to expose the popliteal artery fully. Otherwise, the popliteal artery is dissected free, isolated, and controlled exactly as described for the medial approach.

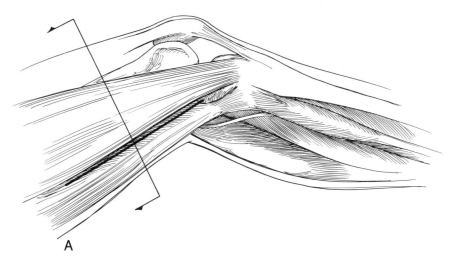

A

Figure 76

A, The incision for lateral exposure of the popliteal artery is placed over the palpable groove between the vastus lateralis and the biceps femoris. *B,* A cross-sectional view of the route taken shows it stays high, just behind the femur, to avoid the popliteal vein that lies lateral and inferior to it. *C,* The dense fascia lata, which bars entry to the popliteal space, must be widely opened by cruciate incisions at each end or *excision* of a generous swath of fascia. *D,* When mobilized through use of traction on encircling loops, the popliteal artery can be brought up into the wound enough to perform an anastomosis comfortably.

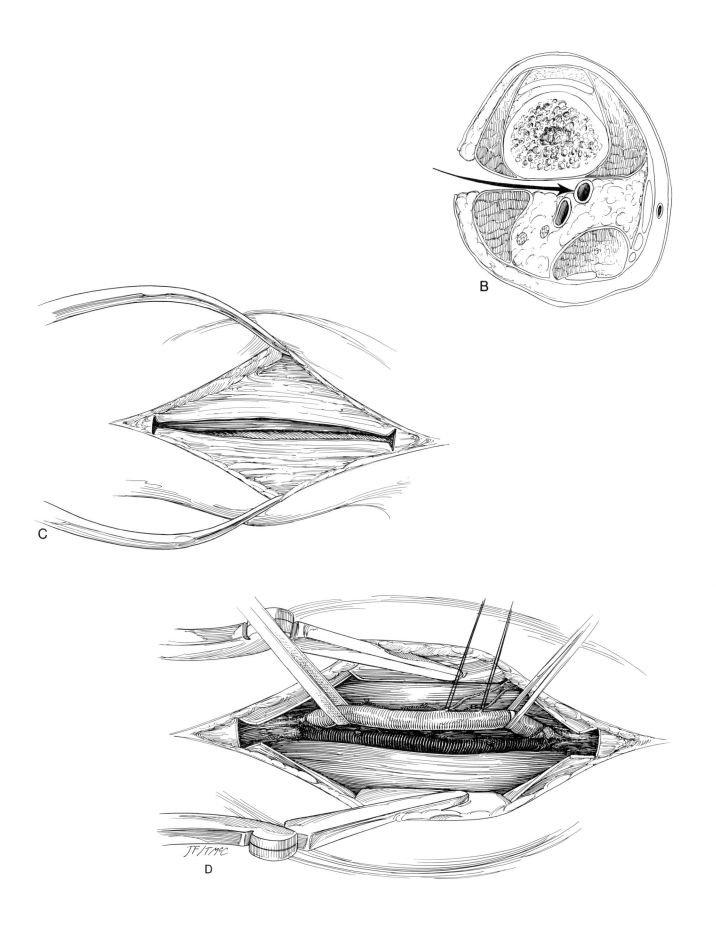

B

C

D

JF/TMC

Vascular Exposures

Posterior Approach to the Popliteal Vessels
(Incision G; Fig. 67)

This is the preferred approach for popliteal artery entrapment and popliteal artery cysts, as well as some midpopliteal artery aneurysms that are of limited extent and/or require complete exposure, evacuation, or segmental *excision,* as in ruptured or infected aneurysms or those producing nerve or vein compression. In addition, in focal midpopliteal trauma, as might be associated with posterior knee dislocation, this approach has merit. Occasionally, it may serve as the proximal end of a *lesser* saphenous in situ bypass to a tibial or pedal artery, usually in patients with diabetes. In most other situations, combining the above- and below-knee medial approaches, detaching muscles to the degree required, is preferable and provides more extensile exposure. Rehabilitation after this posterior approach is *not* necessarily faster or better tolerated than with the combination of medial approaches, because this posterior wound tends to become more swollen, possibly owing to divided lymphatics and superficial veins, and because incisional discomfort may be more bothersome when the knee is flexed, while walking or sitting.

To obtain posterior exposure, a midcalf vertical incision is acutely curved medially just below the popliteal crease, then sharply curved upward again along the posteromedial aspect of the thigh within a centimeter or two of the course of the greater saphenous vein (see Fig. 77A). This incision allows ready access to the greater or lesser saphenous veins, if an autograft or vein patch is required; avoids traversing the popliteal crease in the midline behind the knee; and provides good extensile exposure of the popliteal vessels.

The route into the popliteal vessels is direct (Fig. 77B), passing deeply *medial* to the lesser saphenous vein and sural nerve and to the popliteal vein and its tributaries, as one proceeds between the two heads of the gastrocnemius muscle. With the superficial dissection, care must be taken to avoid injury, not only to the lesser saphenous vein but to the accompanying sural nerve as well. When the gastrocnemius muscles are retracted to each side, one will encounter a nerve branch to the medial head, which may be difficult to preserve if extended exposure is needed (Fig. 77C). In most older patients, its division produces no noticeable disability. One or two tributaries of the popliteal vein will require division before mobilizing the popliteal artery, with the venae comitantes being handled as described previously for the medial above-knee approach. The final exposure shown (Fig. 77D) is primarily of the midpopliteal artery, but this can be extended proximally and distally (with the skin and fascia incisions extended as needed) to reach from just below the adductor hiatus to the origin of the anterior tibial artery.

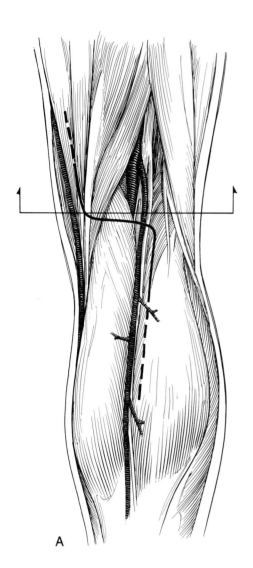

A

Figure 77

A, Stepped incision for posterior exposure of the popliteal vessels is shown, which allows more extensile exposure and access to either greater or lesser saphenous vein grafts, while avoiding perpendicular crossing of the crease. *B,* The route to the popliteal artery, between the two heads of the gastrocnemius muscle, stays *medial* to the sural and posterior tibial nerves and the lesser saphenous and popliteal veins. *C,* A view of the popliteal artery in the depths of the wound, with the accompanying vein and posterior tibial nerve lateral to it. Only popliteal venous tributaries, venae comitantes, and a nerve twig to the medial head of the gastrocnemius bar the way. *D,* With mobilization and retraction of the popliteal vein and the nerve to the medial head of the gastrocnemius muscle, the popliteal artery is isolated and encircled with tapes.

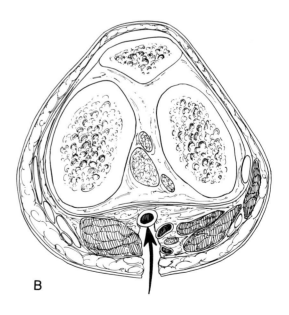

B

Vascular Exposures

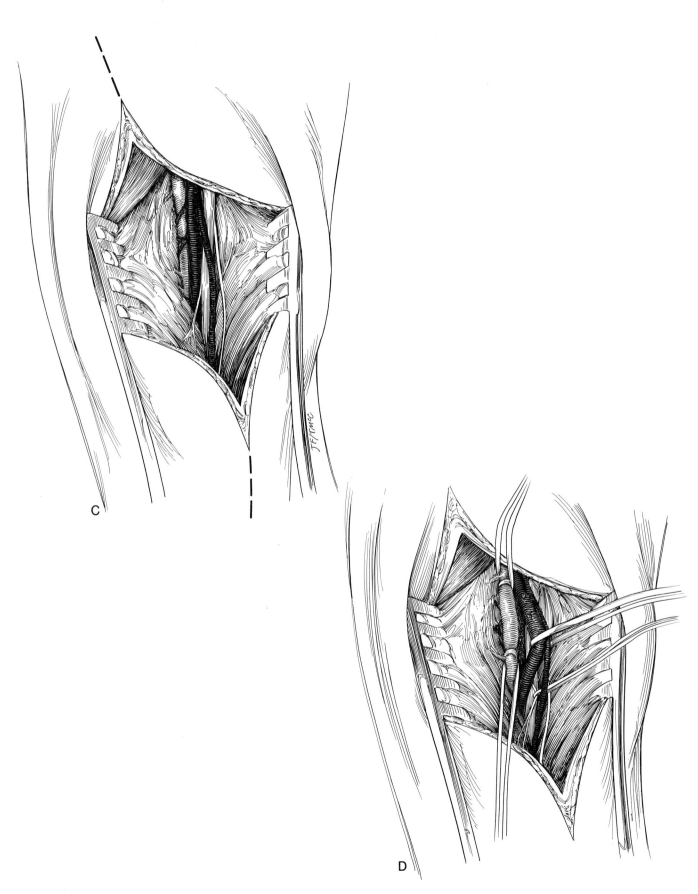

C

D

Infragenicular Exposures

Exposures that are most commonly used in bypass surgery are shown in Figure 68 and labeled from H to P on the medial and lateral aspects of the lower leg and feet. Usually, the knee will be slightly flexed and the leg externally rotated for medial incisions. The allowable degree of internal rotation is so limited that, for laterally placed incisions, the knee is flexed as needed, held in internal rotation, and then the entire patient (actually, the operating table) is tilted away from the operating surgeon (who stands laterally) to allow the first assistant to work effectively. Tilting the patient's pelvis slightly to one side or the other, during the initial positioning, will help only if all the incisions are on the same side (i.e., either on the medial or lateral aspect of the lower extremity). Unfortunately, with laterally placed bypasses one usually still has to harvest the greater saphenous vein medially.

Medial Exposure of the Infragenicular Popliteal Artery and its Branches (Incision H; Fig. 68)

This may be the second most common lower extremity arterial exposure, after that of the femoral artery, being the preferred termination of femoropopliteal artery bypass when utilizing a greater saphenous vein graft. As seen in Figure 78A, the longitudinal incision begins at the level of the knee joint just posterior to the medial condyle of the femur, and runs a fingerbreadth behind the posteromedial edge of the tibia and approximately an equal distance anterior to the usual course of the greater saphenous vein. This allows the latter to be briefly inspected for true size before proceeding with the popliteal artery exposure and provides early assurance of adequate diameter, for it may go into spasm later during the popliteal exposure.

The cross-sectional view (Fig. 78B) shows the correct route into the popliteal vessels, after division of the fascia and the upper soleus muscle as needed. It can be seen here that the popliteal vessels are quite deep and, in fact, are located equidistant from the lateral and medial aspects of the leg.

Once the skin incision is made and the greater saphenous vein inspected, the fascia just behind (posterior to) the tibia is incised (Fig. 78C). With adequate retraction, the popliteal vessels can usually be seen in the depths of the wound superiorly, but inferiorly they are covered to a variable degree by the upper origin of the soleus muscle on the tibia (inset, Fig. 78C). Therefore, for adequate popliteal vessel exposure, division of the upper fibers of the soleus muscle is usually necessary. This is best accomplished with cautery (Fig. 78D), while being aware of an annoying soleal vein tributary that typically exits from the upper aspect of this muscle.

As seen in Figure 78E, when the underlying popliteal vessels are fully visualized, the vein lies over the artery in the lower aspect of the incision—that is, from approximately the level of the anterior tibial artery origin distally. How best to mobilize the vein to expose the artery adequately depends on which end of the arterial segment one wishes to operate on. Thus, if one wishes to gain access to the popliteal artery more proximally and only down as far as the level of the anterior tibial origin, the vein is better retracted downward (posteriorly). This *may* require division of the anterior tibial vein, particularly if the origin of the anterior tibial artery is to be exposed, mobilized, and controlled. This exposure

Vascular Exposures

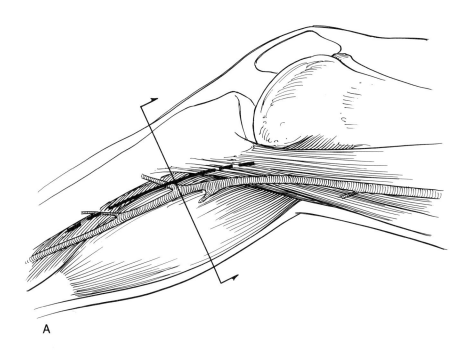

A

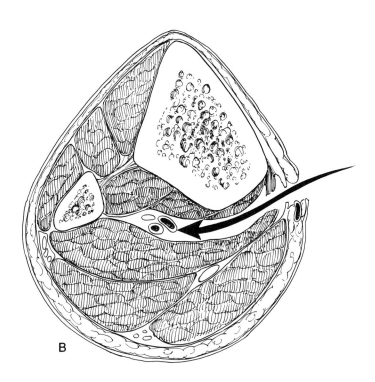

B

Figure 78

A, For medial exposure of the infragenicular popliteal artery, the incision is placed just below the edge of the tibia and in front of the course of the greater saphenous vein. *B,* The route into the popliteal vessels, through the fascia into the deep posterior compartment, with only the soleus muscle partially barring the way. *C,* The fascia is opened, after first inspecting the greater saphenous vein, allowing the popliteal vessels to be seen in the depths of the wound, partially obscured by the upper fibers of the soleus muscle (see inset). *D,* The upper portion of the overlying soleus muscle is divided by cautery. *E,* With retraction of the divided soleus, the popliteal vein is encountered, with the posterior tibial nerve adjacent to it superiorly and slightly deeper. The artery is between them and still deeper, but inferiorly it is completely obscured by the overlying vein. *F,* To expose the popliteal artery *superiorly* (above the anterior tibial origin), the vein is retracted *posteriorly*. For full mobilization, the anterior tibial vein may need to be divided. *G,* To expose the *distal* popliteal artery, tibioperoneal trunk, and its two main branches, the popliteal vein is retracted *anteriorly*. For full mobilization, a major venous tributary from the soleal veins may require division.

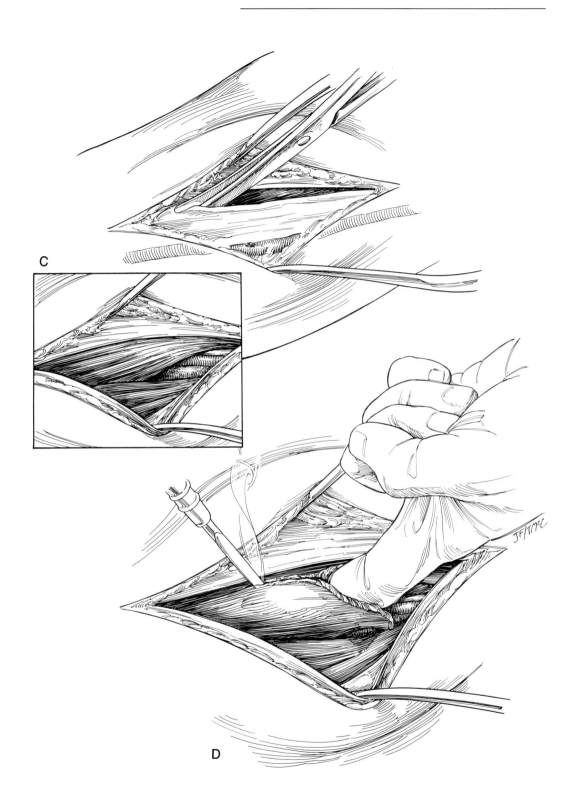

C

D

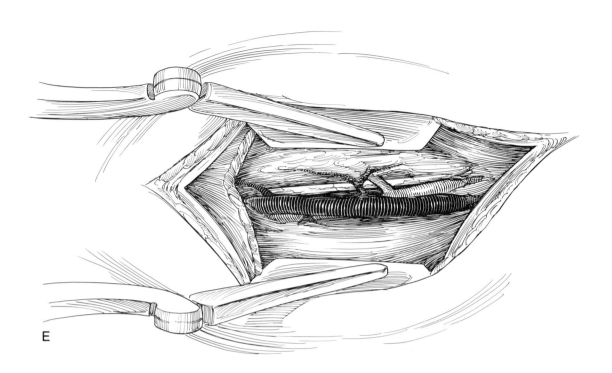

E

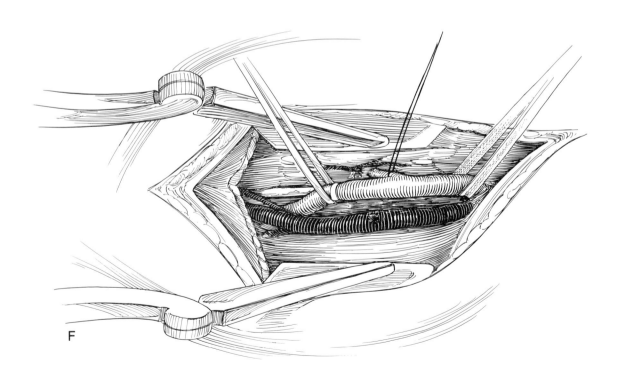

F

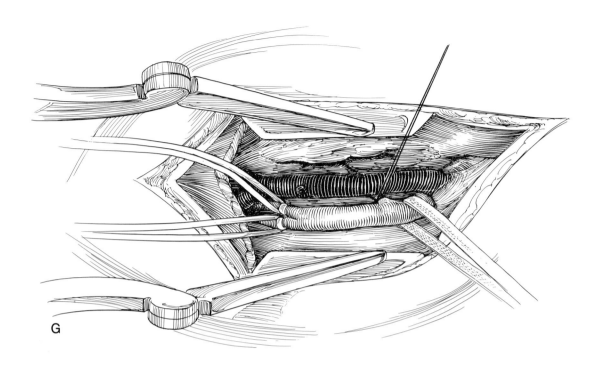

G

is shown in Figure 78*F*. In this regard, it should be noted that upward mobilization of the anterior tibial artery is best achieved by first applying traction to encircling tapes placed around the popliteal artery and the tibioperoneal trunk above and below this level, respectively. The anterior tibial artery location may not be immediately apparent and it may seem to be buried somewhere in the depths of the wound. However, its location can be determined by applying upward traction at different points along the popliteal artery and noting the level at which this segment is most tethered down. Full mobilization of the proximal 2 cm of the anterior tibial artery will be facilitated by opening the interosseus membrane, but this must be done carefully because of small veins in this area that can cause annoying bleeding. Furthermore, this much mobilization is not necessary if one wishes to control only back bleeding from the anterior tibial artery. This can be achieved by traction on proximal and distal tapes while the origin of the anterior tibial is doubly encircled with a Potts loop.

If the tibioperoneal trunk and its branches, the peroneal and posterior tibial arteries, are the focus of attention, the popliteal vein should be mobilized upward (anteriorly). This will require division of a major posterior tributary and result in the exposure shown in Figure 78*G*. During both of these dissections, cautery must be used with great caution for the posterior tibial nerve lies anteriorly, alongside the vein, and in front of the artery (Fig. 78*E* and *F*). Although the aforementioned applies to the usual anatomy, duplication of the popliteal vein is not uncommon.

Vascular Exposures

Lateral Approach to the Below-Knee Popliteal Artery (Incision I; Fig. 68)

This approach is particularly useful if an operation has previously been performed from the medial side because returning through that approach is often complicated by a combination of scar tissue *and* an overlying vein, and venous bleeding may be extremely vexing. It is also useful in popliteal-distal bypasses to laterally placed arteries, most commonly performed in diabetic patients.

As shown in Figure 79*A*, the incision begins just behind the head of the fibula and continues along its course about one-quarter the distance to the lateral malleolus. The route into the popliteal vessels is barred by the fibula (Fig. 79*B*), which fortunately is expendable in elderly patients, particularly if only a segment is removed subperiosteally. In time, the defect will usually bridge over completely. Thus, the initial approach involves cleaning off the lateral surface of the upper fibula. Of critical importance here is the location of the superficial peroneal nerve, which curves around the upper fibula, just below its head, from posterior to anterior. It may or may not be visualized and gently retracted (Fig. 79*C*), but exposure and division of the periosteum over the fibula should begin distally and proceed proximally with caution. Staying inside the periosteum will ordinarily ensure the nerve is mobilized upward and anteriorly with other tissues. The periosteum is then elevated circumferentially around the fibula for the length of the incision; the exposed segment is then excised, after drilling two holes through it, using a rib shear (Fig. 79*C*). After this, the underlying periosteum is incised and the vessels are found directly beneath it, with the vein fortunately located *behind* the artery (Fig. 79*D*). After mobilizing the artery from accompanying veins and exposing and controlling the distal popliteal artery, the origins of the anterior tibial and the tibioperoneal trunk are exposed and controlled with Silastic loops (Fig. 79*E*). By "lowering" the incision appropriately (by placing or extending it more distally and/or removing more fibula), the tibioperoneal trunk and its branches can also be exposed through this approach.

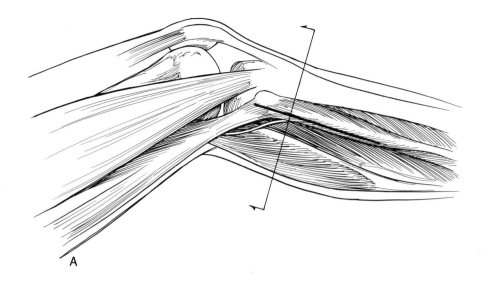

A

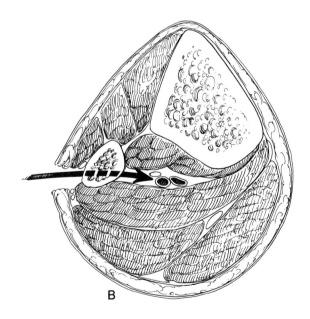

Figure 79

A, For lateral exposure of the infragenicular popliteal vessels, the incision is placed over the upper fibula. *B,* Cross-sectional view shows the popliteal vessel lying on a soleal sling behind the fibula.

B

Vascular Exposures

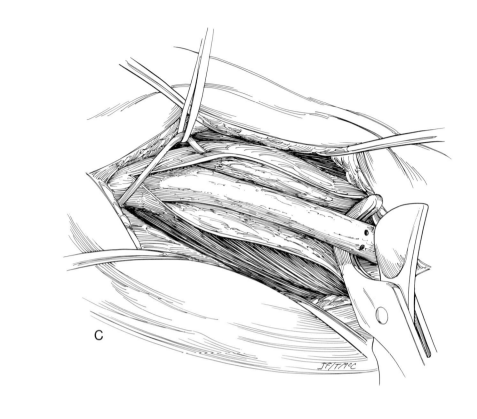

C

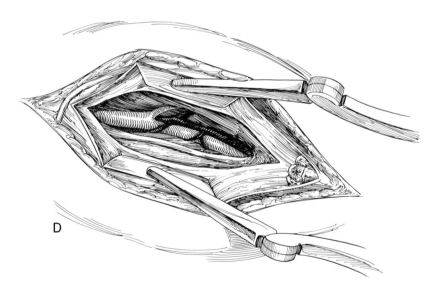

D

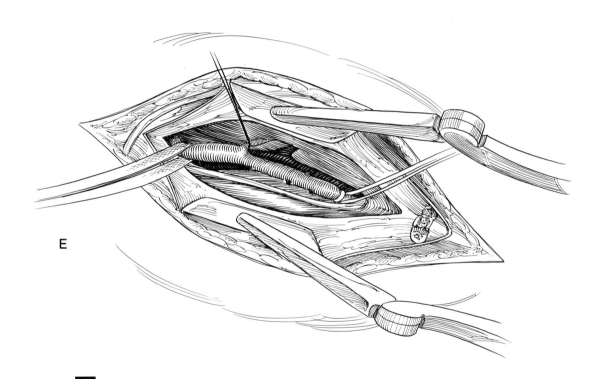

E

Figure 79 *Continued*

C, The upper fibula is removed subperiosteally. Only rarely is the superficial peroneal nerve visualized and retracted, as shown here to emphasize its location and proximity to injury. *D,* When the deep fibular periosteum is incised, the popliteal vessels are seen just beyond, above the posterior tibial nerve and in front of the popliteal vein. *E,* After it is freed from venae comitantes, the popliteal artery and its branches are encircled with tapes.

Vascular Exposures

Medial Approach to the Posterior Tibial Artery at the Ankle (Incision J; Fig. 68)

If the upper posterior tibial artery is not patent, the next most frequent location where it is exposed is just above the ankle, where it is not only more accessible but also beyond much of the occlusive disease that potentially may involve it. This incision also provides a good location for in situ bypass, with the greater saphenous vein being conveniently located nearby. The incision may be made halfway between the malleolus and the Achilles tendon, or slightly more anterior if in situ bypass is planned (Fig. 80A). A Doppler probe often locates the patent but pulseless distal artery (or the adjacent vein), and this can be used to guide the placement of the incision. Once the fascia is opened, the neurovascular bundle is usually easily located in a fatty envelope separate from adjacent muscles and tendons. The vein is most readily seen as the perivascular fat is dissected away. The artery usually lies more anterior and deeper than the vein with the nerve more posterior (Fig. 80B). Venae comitantes are usually numerous but can be dissected away with care to isolate and control an adequate length of artery (Fig. 80C).

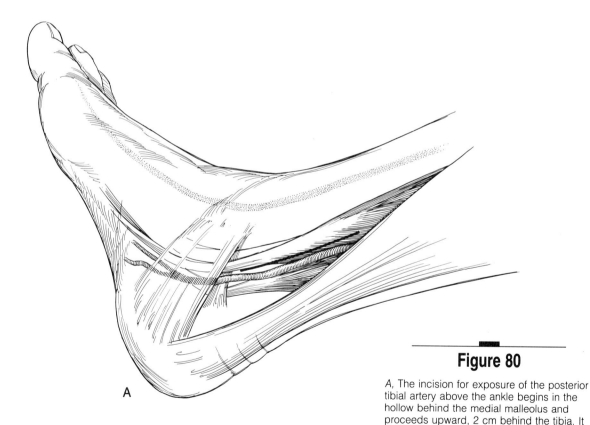

A

Figure 80

A, The incision for exposure of the posterior tibial artery above the ankle begins in the hollow behind the medial malleolus and proceeds upward, 2 cm behind the tibia. It may be moved anteriorly to allow concomitant exposure of the greater saphenous vein (shaded outline) before their courses diverge. B, When the fascia is opened, the neurovascular bundle is found surrounded by fat. The artery is usually superior with the nerve inferior. C, The posterior tibial artery is isolated and controlled with tapes.

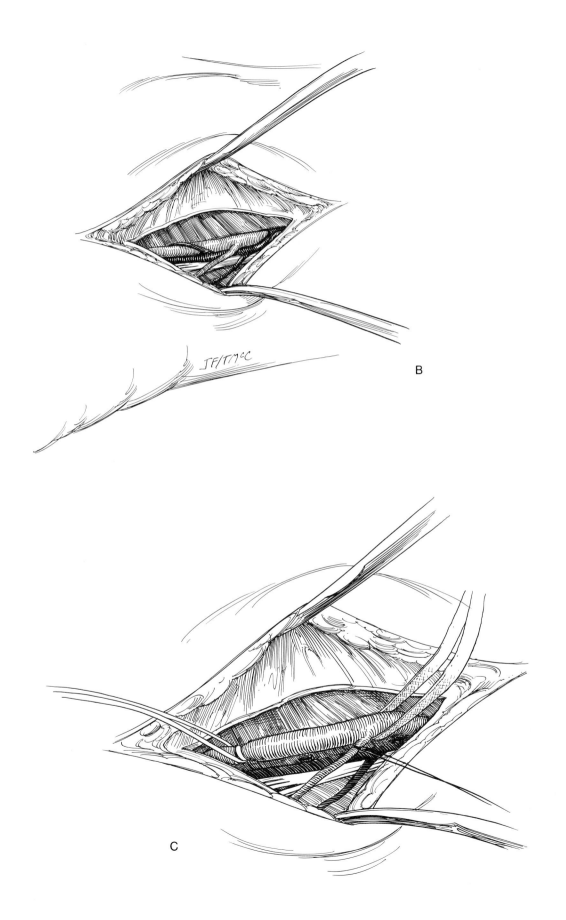

B

C

Vascular Exposures

Exposure of the Middle Segment of the Posterior Tibial Artery (Incision K; Fig. 68)

The main reason to choose this intermediate segment is limited length of vein graft. From the upper posterior tibial artery to its supramalleolar segment, the only major intervening structure is the soleus muscle. Preferably, exposure of the middle segment of the posterior tibial artery should be obtained just below the midpoint where the soleus is thin or absent (Fig. 81*A*). At this point, the greater saphenous vein is even closer to an incision over the artery than just above the malleolus, so that in situ bypass is easily performed here. As shown in Figure 81*B*, this exposure allows an approach that is midway in depth between the proximal and distal segment exposures and, once the lower edge of the covering soleus muscle is divided by cautery (Fig. 81*C*), the underlying vessels are soon encountered (Fig. 81*D*). Usually, the accompanying vein lies superiorly, with the nerve posterior to the artery. Final exposure of the posterior tibial artery is shown in Figure 81*E*. Although the peroneal artery is much deeper, it can also be reached through this incision by retracting the posterior tibial vessels downward and dissecting deeper in the cleft between the soleus and tibialis posterior muscles (cross section, Fig. 81*B*).

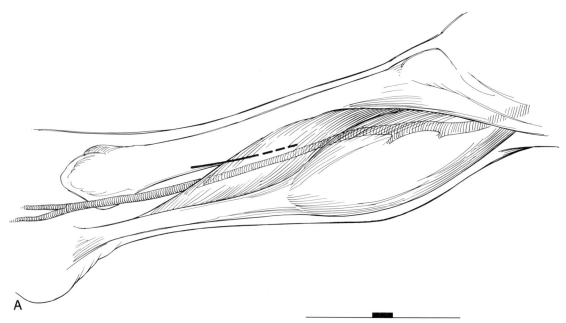

A

Figure 81

A, Medial exposure of the middle segment of the posterior tibial artery is best accomplished at or below the lower edge of the soleus muscle. *B,* Cross section shows the route to the posterior tibial vessels, anterior to the gastrocnemius muscle with the peroneal vessels further lateral. *C,* Division of the lower fibers of the soleus muscle. The nerve is gently retracted out of harm's way.

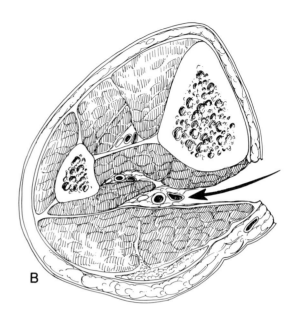

B

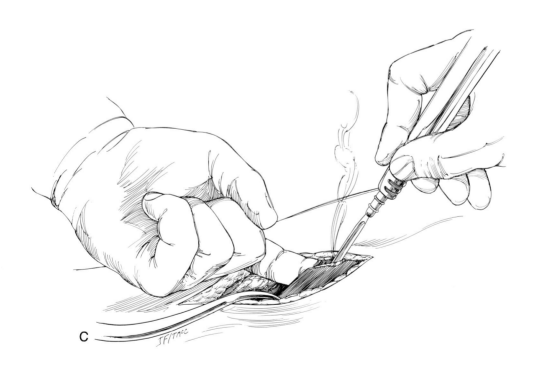

C

Vascular Exposures

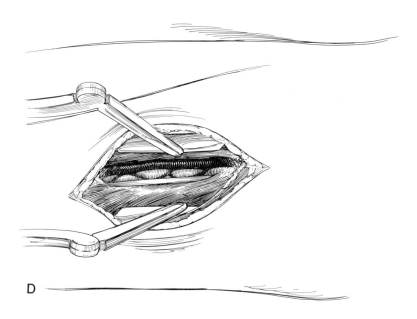

D

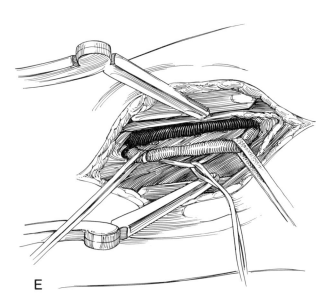

E

Figure 81 *Continued*

D, Exposure of the posterior tibial artery with the vein above and the nerve below. *E*, Final exposure after dividing venae comitantes and mobilizing the artery.

Anterolateral Approach to the Proximal Anterior Tibial Artery (Incision L; Fig. 68)

The proximal centimeter or two of the anterior tibial artery is a site of predilection for atheromatous disease, possibly related to its more perpendicular takeoff and its passage through the intermuscular septum. Beyond this it is often relatively disease free and readily accessible through an anterolateral approach. The incision for exposing the upper third is placed in a vertical plane about 2 FB lateral to the anterior edge of the tibia (Fig. 82A). The cross-sectional view (Fig. 82B) shows that the anterior vessels lie on or near the intermuscular septum, at the bottom of a valley formed by the tibialis anterior and the extensor hallucis longus muscles. When the muscles are not atrophied, this cleft is narrow and requires strong, deep, self-retaining retractors, like Ochsner's. Here, small vessels rise up from the posterior tibial vessels to enter the muscles on either side (Fig. 82C). They are easily torn by retractors or blunt dissection. The anterior tibial vein often overlies the artery and venae comitantes are numerous and particularly vexing if torn. The ensuing trouble is well worth avoiding by carefully dissecting them free and ligating and dividing them wherever they bar the way to the anterior tibial artery. They are more easily dealt with if the thin, membranous overlying sheath is first carefully incised. Magnification is very helpful here, as it is with most tibial exposures and anastomoses. Once the overlying veins are dealt with, the artery is readily isolated and controlled (Fig. 82D). By extending the incision, or placing it farther distally (see dotted line between incisions L and M in Figure 68), the anterior tibial can be exposed where there is less muscle to retract and the incision is shallower. However, this requires a longer graft and the artery will be somewhat smaller in diameter as one proceeds distally.

Vascular Exposures

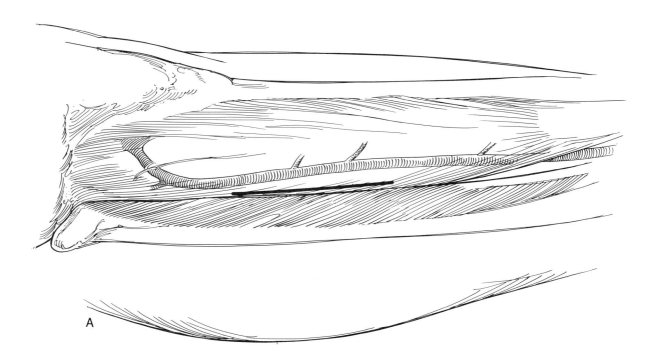

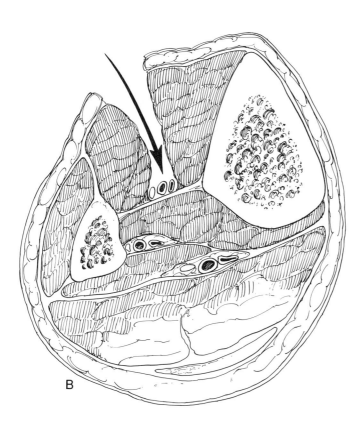

Figure 82

A, The location of incision for exposure of the upper anterior tibial artery. *B,* Cross-sectional view showing the anterior tibial vessels lying on the interosseus membrane, and the route to them between the tibialis anterior and the extensor hallucis longus muscles. *C,* The anterior tibial artery, surrounded with venae comitantes, with lateral twigs to adjacent muscles. *D,* Exposure requires careful dissection away from overlying venae comitantes, which require ligation and division. [*C* and *D* are viewed from the medial aspect of the right leg (head to the right.)]

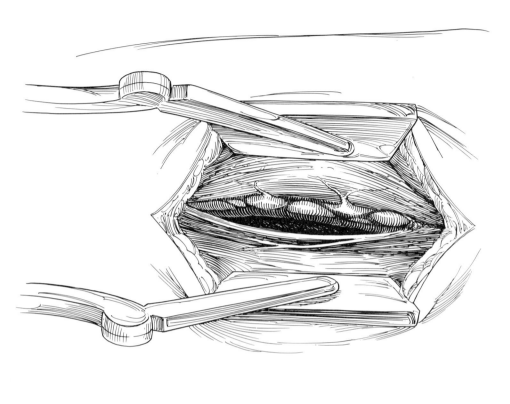

C

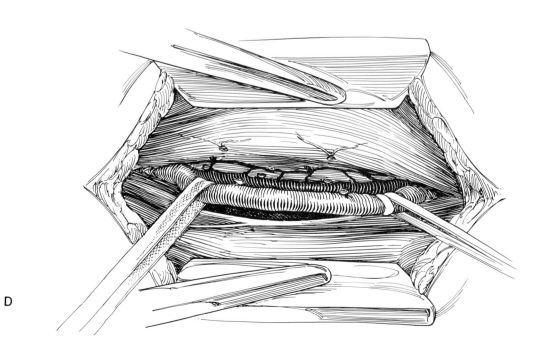

D

Vascular Exposures

*Exposure of the Supramalleolar Anterior Tibial
Artery (Incision M; Fig. 68)*

If the proximal third of the anterior tibial artery is not suitable, and vein length is not a consideration, it is usually best to expose the artery just above the ankle and the flexor retinaculum because this area usually is less involved with disease, quite superficial, and more easily reached for in situ bypass (Fig. 83*A*). It is also surrounded by tendons. Normally, the best route passes between the extensor hallucis longus and the extensor digitorum longus laterally and the extensor hallucis brevis and tibialis anterior medially (see cross section, Fig. 83*B*). Once these tendons are retracted, the artery is readily found, exposed, and isolated after dealing with vena comitantes and branches of the anterior tibial vein (Fig. 83*C*).

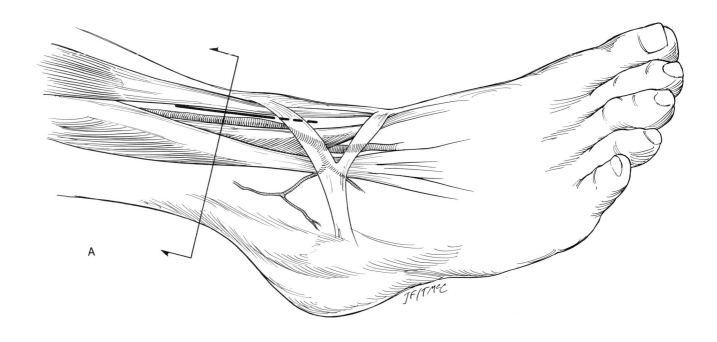

A

Figure 83

A, Incision for exposure of the anterior tibial artery just above the ankle, where it is surrounded by tendons coursing under the upper extensor retinaculum. *B*, Cross section shows the anterior tibial vessels lying just above the periosteum of the tibia between the tendons of the tibialis anterior and extensor hallucis longus. *C*, With retraction of the tendons, exposure is not difficult, although the upper extensor retinaculum may need to be divided for lower exposure.

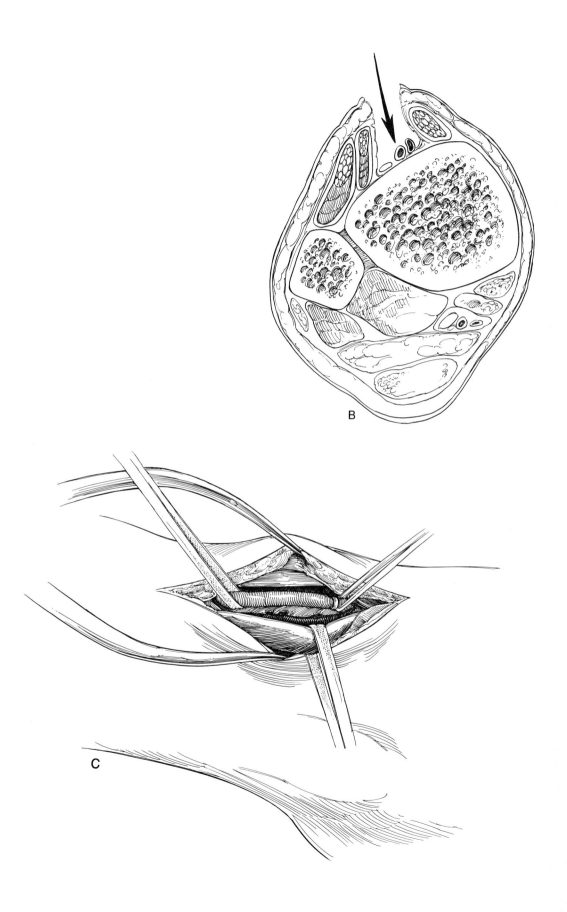

B

C

Vascular Exposures

Lateral Approach to the Peroneal Artery (Incision N; Fig. 68)

Exposure of the proximal peroneal artery can be obtained as an extension of exposure of the distal popliteal artery, either medially or laterally, as described previously. It can also be exposed in its midportion from a medial approach, continuing past the posterior tibial artery, using incision K in Figure 68. However, in the author's experience, the easiest exposure is one that might seem, at first, more difficult (i.e., approaching it laterally, through the bed of an excised segment of fibula). This is a natural extension of the lateral approach to the distal popliteal artery, but it is considerably easier.

The incision is made vertically over the fibula at the desired level, selected by inspection of the arteriogram (Fig. 84A). Once the thin overlying muscle is dissected away, arterial exposure requires only segmental fibular resection and incision of the underlying fascia (Fig. 84B). Once the periosteum of the fibula has been completely elevated circumferentially, two holes are drilled at either end at the proposed points of division, to allow the rib shears to achieve a simple transection without comminution (Fig. 84C). Once the fibula is removed, incising the underlying periosteum brings one directly down on the peroneal vessels (Fig. 84D). Freeing the underlying artery requires dissecting it free from the venae comitantes and branches of the peroneal vein (Fig. 84E). A suitably soft segment of artery can be located by gently squeezing the artery with vascular forceps.

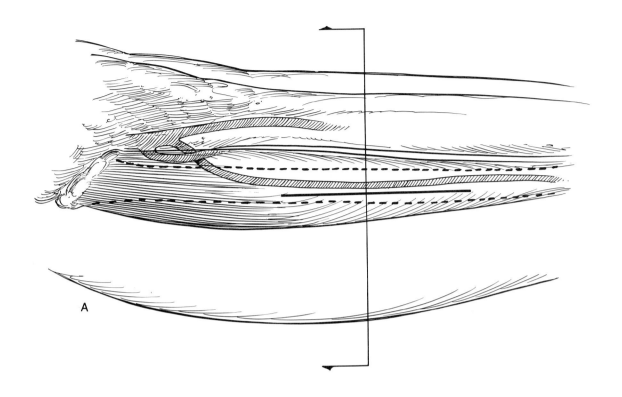

Figure 84

A, Lateral exposure of the peroneal artery requires an incision over the fibula, which is represented by dotted lines, at the level of the most suitably patent segment. *B,* Cross section shows the peroneal vessels lying just below the fibula.

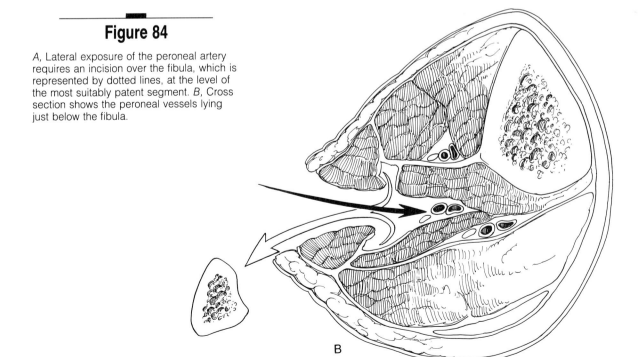

Vascular Exposures

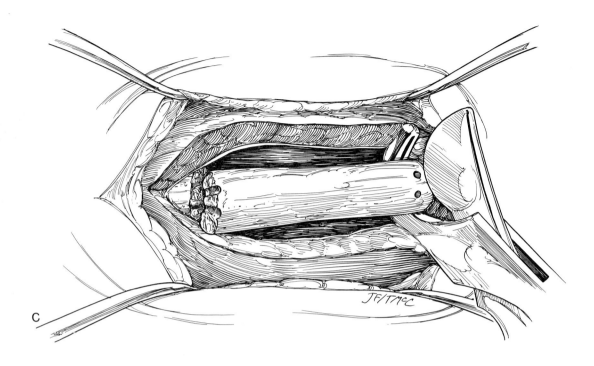

C

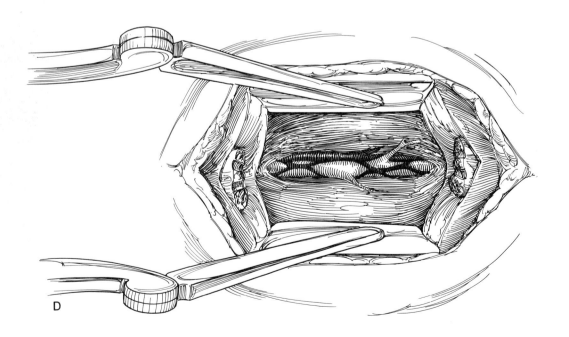

D

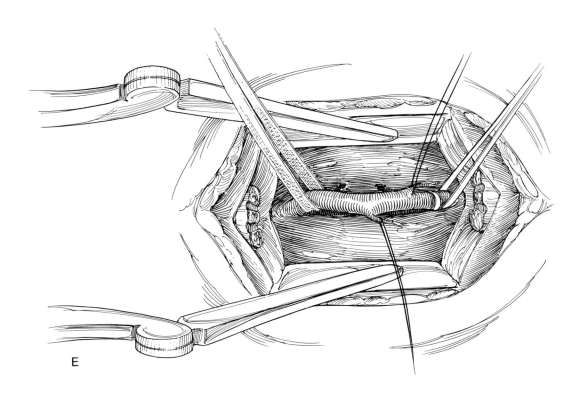

E

Figure 84 *Continued*

C, The overlying fibula is transected more cleanly with rib shears if two holes are first drilled at the desired level. *D*, With the fibular segment excised and its inner periosteal membrane incised, the peroneal vessels are immediately encountered. *E*, Final exposure of the peroneal artery after mobilization from surrounding venae comitantes.

Vascular Exposures

*Exposure of the Inframalleolar Posterior Tibial
Artery and the Lateral Plantar Artery
(Incision O; Fig. 68)*

As pointed out by Veith and Gupta, in patients with diabetes the only patent segment of distal artery may be the posterior tibial artery just proximal to its lateral plantar branch, with outflow extending into the latter vessel itself. Exposure is achieved by using a distal extension of the supramalleolar exposure, following the course of the posterior tibial artery distally and incising the overlying ligament and all or part of the overlying adductor hallucis brevis muscle (Fig. 85A). Here, in a tangle of venae comitantes (Fig. 85B), the "bifurcation" will be found. Depending on the most suitable segment, best detected by gently squeezing the artery with fine forceps, the overlying veins are dissected away and the segment is isolated and controlled (Fig. 85C). To gain adequate length for an anastomosis, it is often started on the distal posterior tibial artery but carried across the origin of the lateral plantar artery and on into that vessel for 0.5 to 1.0 cm.

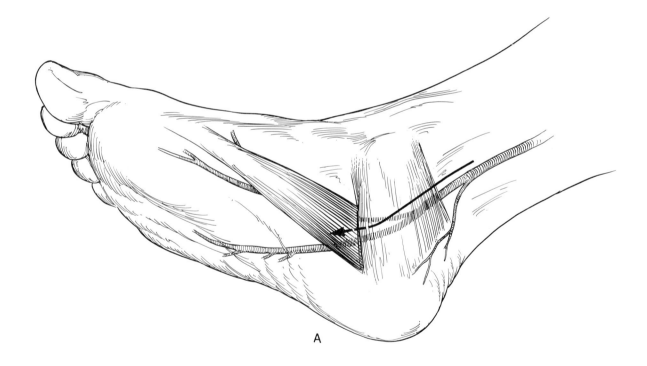

A

Figure 85

A, Exposure of the inframalleolar posterior tibial artery is best achieved by carrying the usual higher incision downward, dividing the overlying flexor retinaculum and, as required, upper fibers of the adductor hallucis brevis. *B,* With these structures divided, the bifurcation of the posterior tibial artery is seen, with surrounding veins and adjacent nerve. *C,* Mobilization of a suitable segment of the distal posterior tibial artery often requires inclusion of the first centimeter of its lateral plantar branch.

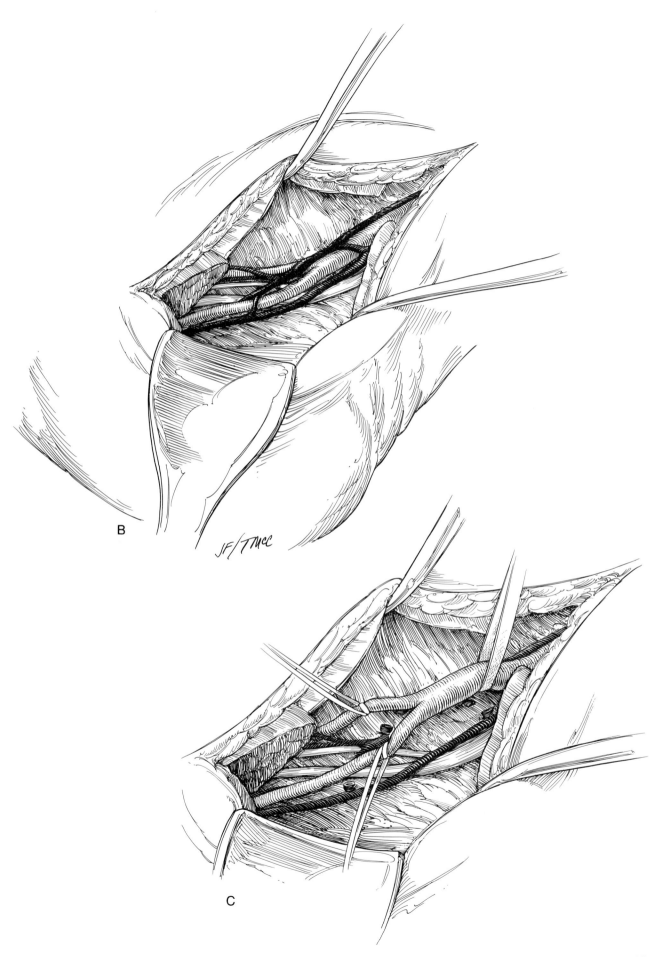

B

JF/TMCC

C

Vascular Exposures

Exposure of the Dorsalis Pedis and Deep Tarsal
Arteries (Incision P; Fig. 68)

Again, usually in patients with diabetes, the pedal extension of the anterior tibial artery may, on occasion, be the only suitable termination for a distal bypass. The incision for this is made from just beyond the extensor retinaculum downward, spanning the space between the first and second metatarsal bones (Fig. 86*A*). The dorsalis pedis vessels and the accompanying nerve will be readily encountered (Fig. 86*B*). A suitable segment, suggested by the arteriogram and confirmed by gently squeezing the vessel, is selected for exposure. Occasionally, this will be found to extend into the deep tarsal branch. To gain additional exposure of that branch, a segment of the second metatarsal bone usually must be resected (Fig. 86*C*). Final exposure is shown in Figure 86*D*.

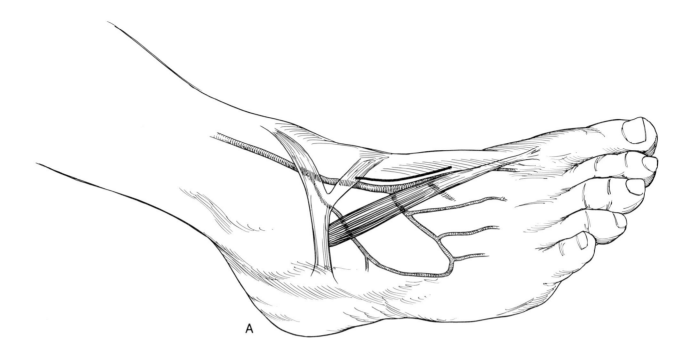

Figure 86

A, Incision to expose the dorsalis pedis artery below the extensor retinaculum courses along a longitudinal line that ends just lateral to the first metatarsal head.

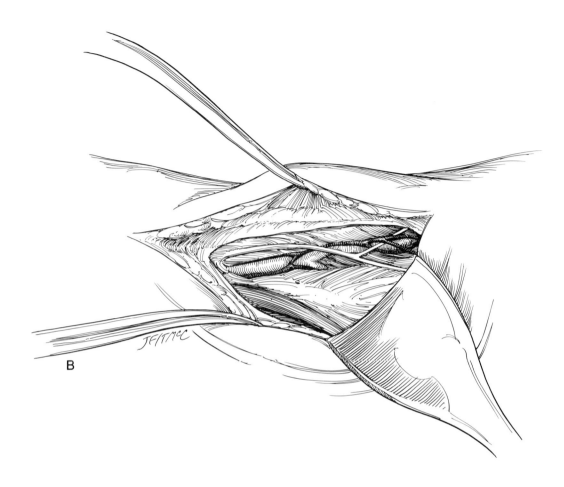

B

Figure 86 *Continued*

B, The dorsalis pedis artery is seen in a
groove between the first and second
metatarsal heads. *C,* Extension into the
medial tarsal branch requires excision of the
proximal second metatarsal bone. *D,* Final
exposure with controlling tapes and loops.

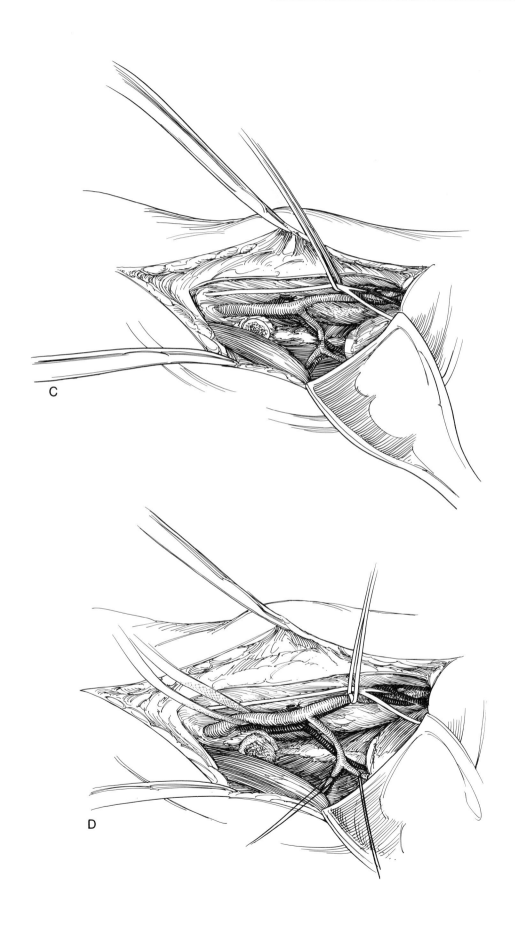

EXPOSURES OF THE AORTA AND ITS MAJOR BRANCHES

Although infrainguinal bypass may be the vascular surgeon's "bread and butter" and its usual origin, the femoral bifurcation, the most common exposure, it is operations on the aorta and its major branches that lead to the surgeon's greatest technical challenges. Infrarenal abdominal aortic exposure is probably second only to femoral artery exposure in frequency. From this central point, one can move downward to the groin in managing aortoiliac occlusive disease, move laterally to revascularize visceral arteries, or move progressively upward to deal with lesions of the suprarenal aorta all the way to the origin of the left subclavian artery. This is also the sequence of exposures described in this subsection.

Exposure of the Infrarenal Aorta

Two of the most common vascular operations, aortic aneurysm repair and aortobifemoral bypass, require exposure of the infrarenal aorta. The most common method utilizes a direct transabdominal approach. This is most frequently carried out through a long midline incision, although a transverse incision is still very popular among individuals trained in certain institutions and is quite acceptable (Fig. 87). Although either one offers adequate exposure of the aorta between the renal arteries and the iliac bifurcation, the midline incision is faster and simpler, whereas the transverse incision causes less pain and should result in fewer pulmonary complications. The increasing use of epidural catheters to control postoperative pain may negate some of the latter's advantage. The author prefers the long midline incision for most situations and, if pulmonary disease and possible pulmonary complications are overriding considerations, a retroperitoneal approach rather than an open transabdominal exposure through a transverse incision is often a better alternative.

Many fail to take advantage of the full extent of the midline incision. The aortic bifurcation is approximately at the level of the umbilicus and therefore exposure of the infrarenal aorta requires that the upper end of the midline incision be extended all the way up to the xiphoid process. If iliac exposure is required, the lower end of the incision should be carried almost to the pubis; otherwise, it may be terminated halfway between the umbilicus and the pubis. The more obese the patient, the longer the incision must be. Aneurysm repairs require greater exposure than a proximal aortic anastomosis to bypass aortoiliac disease. The main advantage of a midline incision is that it may be quickly extended as needed and quickly closed after the operation is completed.

Ordinarily, after the abdomen is opened, a thorough exploration is carried out. Then the transverse colon and greater omentum are drawn up out of the abdomen and draped across the upper operative field, often resting on the lower costal margins. The small intestines are mobilized to the right and, depending on the body habitus and how much gas is in the intestines, they may either be packed off within the abdomen or be eviscerated to obtain adequate exposure. In the eviscerated situation, it is important to keep the bowels covered with moist laparotomy pads and avoid traumatizing them with retractors. If the surgeon stands to the patient's right it helps to rotate the table 10° to 15° toward that side, but many surgeons prefer to approach the aorta standing on the patient's left.

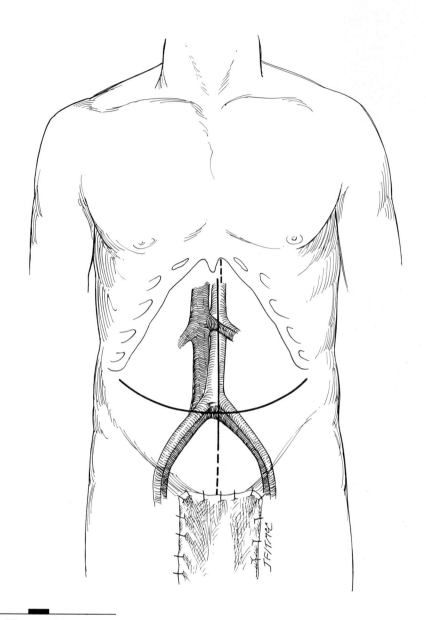

Figure 87

Longitudinal and transverse incisions for
transabdominal approach to the aorta,
inferior vena cava, and iliac vessels. Note
that the bifurcations lie at the level of the
umbilicus.

Vascular Exposures

As shown in Figure 88, after the intestines have been retracted, a longitudinal incision is made along the base of the mesentery. It will be found that the optimum plane to enter (i.e., the one with the least tissue overlying the upper infrarenal aorta between the inferior mesenteric artery and the left renal vein) lies just to the right of the aorta along a vertical line midway between the aorta and the inferior vena cava. The peritoneal layer can be incised along this line with scissors or cautery over a clamp inserted into the underlying areolar tissue and lifted upward to avoid contact with the underlying great vessels. The duodenum lies over the upper infrarenal aorta and ordinarily must be at least partially mobilized to the right. In doing this, the peritoneal incision should be continued upward, staying about 1 cm from the duodenum and leaving a rim of peritoneal reflection to sew to if the duodenum needs to be repositioned.

As one proceeds upward, particularly when approaching the left renal vein, the overlying tissues should be ligated in continuity before division because major mesenteric lymphatics course down through this area to join the cisterna chyli. As the inferior mesenteric vein courses upward, it gradually crosses from left to right over the upper aspect of the infrarenal aorta and, to gain adequate exposure, it may need to be divided, high up, about 2 to 3 cm below its confluence with the splenic vein. This maneuver will often uncover the left renal vein, crossing perpendicularly across the upper infrarenal aorta but in a deeper plane. In fact, the left renal vein should be deliberately sought in that location. A small or absent left renal vein anterior to the aorta may be the only clue (if a preoperative computed tomography [CT] scan has not been obtained) that a retroaortic left renal vein lurks below, a potentially disastrous encounter for the unwary surgeon seeking to gain circumferential proximal aortic control.

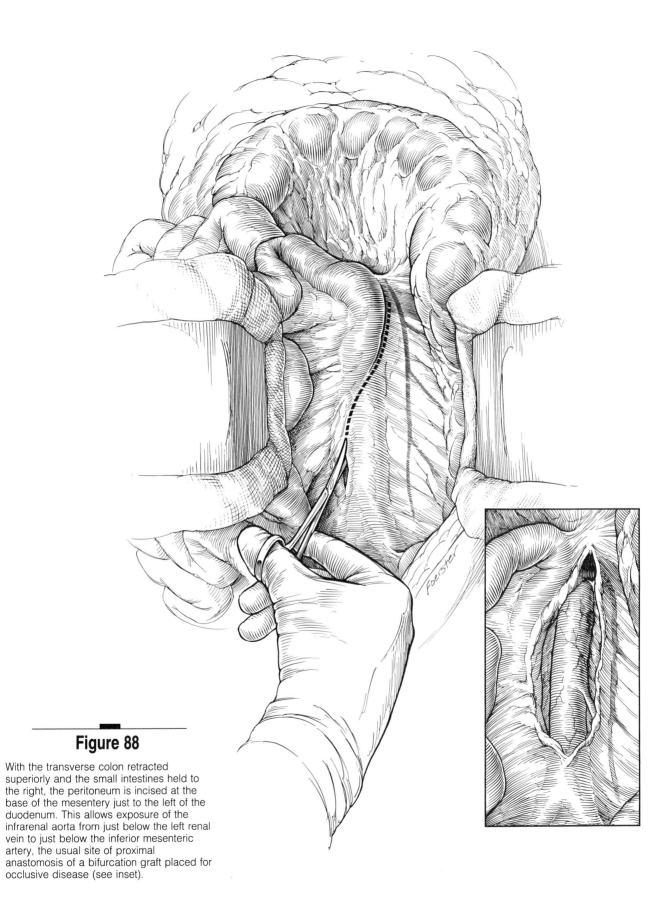

Figure 88

With the transverse colon retracted superiorly and the small intestines held to the right, the peritoneum is incised at the base of the mesentery just to the left of the duodenum. This allows exposure of the infrarenal aorta from just below the left renal vein to just below the inferior mesenteric artery, the usual site of proximal anastomosis of a bifurcation graft placed for occlusive disease (see inset).

Vascular Exposures

In some circumstances, only limited exposure of the infrarenal aorta may be needed; for example, the segment from the left renal vein above to just beyond the inferior mesenteric artery below, as shown in Figure 88 (inset). Ordinarily, this is the ideal segment in which to place the proximal anastomosis of a bifurcation graft. More complete exposure of the infrarenal aorta, as required in dealing with aneurysmal disease, is shown in Figure 89. Here, after visualizing the left renal vein above, one proceeds distally to just beyond the aortic bifurcation, incising the peritoneum over the upper iliac arteries. Figure 89 also shows that the periaortic sympathetic fibers join connecting fibers from the lumbar chains on either side of the aorta to course over the left side of the aortic bifurcation and the origin of the left common iliac artery as they descend into the pelvis, connecting there with the lumbosacral plexus. These will not ordinarily be disturbed in opening the overlying peritoneum but will be injured in carrying an incision in the distal aorta on into the left common iliac artery. This must be avoided in sexually active males to avoid producing retrograde ejaculation and even impotence. Disjointed or step incisions can be used to spare this pathway, and one can work under the preserved bridge of tissue to the left of the bifurcation in performing endarterectomy or tunneling a bypass graft, as pointed out by Machleder.

The basic exposure shown in Figure 89 is adequate for abdominal aortic aneurysm repairs when there is a substantial infrarenal "neck" and no significant iliac artery involvement, that is, conditions permitting placement of a straight or tube graft. For higher exposures (see upper inset in Fig. 89), the left renal vein can be carefully exposed and divided *medially* so that venous inflow from the left kidney can be diverted retrograde through its adrenal, gonadal, and descending lumbar tributaries. Occasionally, if these tributaries have already been divided or are not well developed, as in some children, significant hypertension of the left renal vein will persist and impair renal function, but this is quite uncommon. Nevertheless, it is wise to anticipate this possibility and use the degree of distension in the proximal vein following trial occlusion with a looped ligature to determine whether ligature is safe or not. If not, vascular clamps may be applied before division to allow later anastomosis. Fortunately, the first situation usually pertains and the vein can be ligated with heavy sutures or its end oversewn, with the closure being reinforced with a suture ligature or metal clips, in deference to the 10 to 12 percent of venous return to the heart that must be stemmed. The aorta up to the renal arteries, which lie just above this level, can then be exposed. Then, the origin of the superior mesenteric artery is only a fingerbreadth away anteriorly. This, and the body of the pancreas, restrict higher exposures of the aorta without medial visceral rotation (shown in Fig. 94).

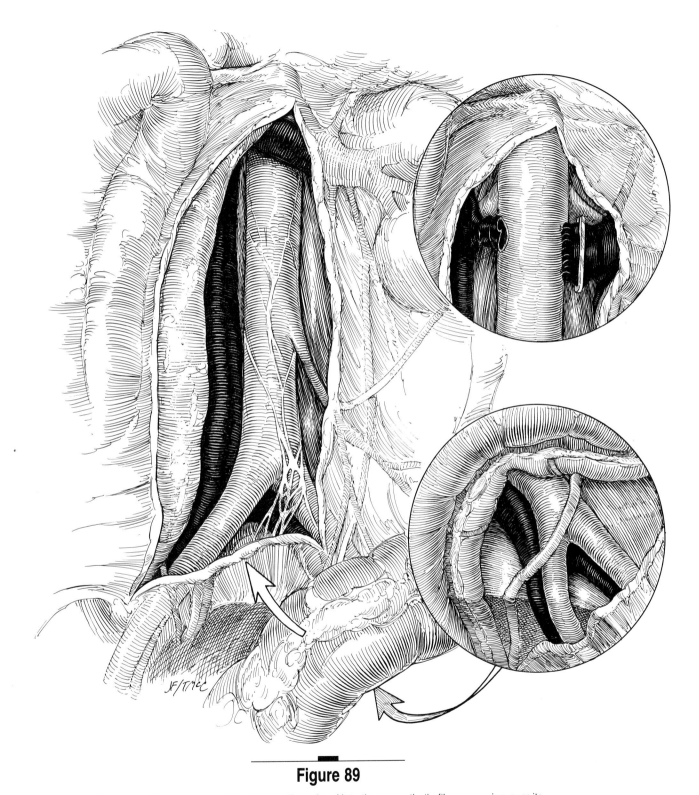

Figure 89

Exposure of the infrarenal aorta and its bifurcation. Note the sympathetic fibers coursing over its anterior surface, communicating with lumbar ganglia laterally and coalescing to travel across the origin of the left common iliac artery and then downward to join the pelvic plexuses. This exposure usually suffices for infrarenal aortic aneurysms. For higher exposure the left renal vein can normally be safely divided medial to its major tributaries (see upper inset showing alternative approaches to secure closure of the divided ends). The left iliac bifurcation cannot be readily exposed and controlled by extension of the aortic incision, as it can on the right. Instead, the rectosigmoid is reflected medially and a counterincision made laterally, providing full exposure (see lower inset).

Vascular Exposures

Exposure of the Iliac Arteries

If further distal exposure down to the iliac artery bifurcations is required, it can be easily obtained on the right by incising the peritoneum over the right iliac artery, retracting the ureter out of the way, but on the left side the sigmoid colon and its mesentery are in the way. Some proximal exposure of the left common iliac is possible before encountering the sigmoid mesentery, as shown in the main illustration in Figure 89. If exposure of the *left* iliac bifurcation is desired, it is usually better to move to the other side of the rectosigmoid colon, making a counterincision laterally along the lower line of Toldt and carrying it down into the pelvis. By staying in the loose areolar tissue plane over the iliopsoas muscles and sweeping the sigmoid mesentery and ureter to the right and upward, the iliac bifurcation will be readily seen and mobilized (as shown in the bottom inset in Fig. 89). With the mesentery retracted upward, a passage beneath it, under the mesenteric vessels but above the ureter, can be bluntly dissected and secured with a large Penrose drain, which facilitates retraction and later passage of the left limb of a bypass graft. The exposure shown in Figure 89, with potential upward extension to the renal arteries and downward extension to allow exposure of the iliac arteries as shown in the two insets, is sufficient for the usual aortoiliac bypass or reconstruction. For aortofemoral bypass, only the proximal exposure shown in Figure 88 (inset) is required, with the graft limbs being tunneled under the peritoneum all the way to the groins from there.

Figure 90A shows a different view of these iliac artery exposures. Parts or all of the incision lines shown might be used if one has already obtained direct transabdominal exposure but is primarily interested in exposure of one or the other iliac arteries, as in endarterectomy or isolated iliac aneurysm repair. Here, after incising the overlying peritoneum, a finger can be inserted into the loose areolar tissue plane directly anterior to the common iliac artery and, with the fingernail intermittently in contact with this surface, the fingertip can be progressively insinuated down this "free" plane to the iliac bifurcation and beyond by repeatedly flexing the distal phalanx, much as in beckoning, thereby progressively elevating the overlying tissue, including the ureter and its accompanying blood supply (inset, Fig. 90A). Then, using counterpressure with the thumb, most of the overlying fatty tissue can be squeezed to one side, leaving the ureter and accompanying vessels visualized and readily protected. In the final exposure (Fig. 90B), the ureter can be retracted either way, depending on which iliac segment is to be accessed.

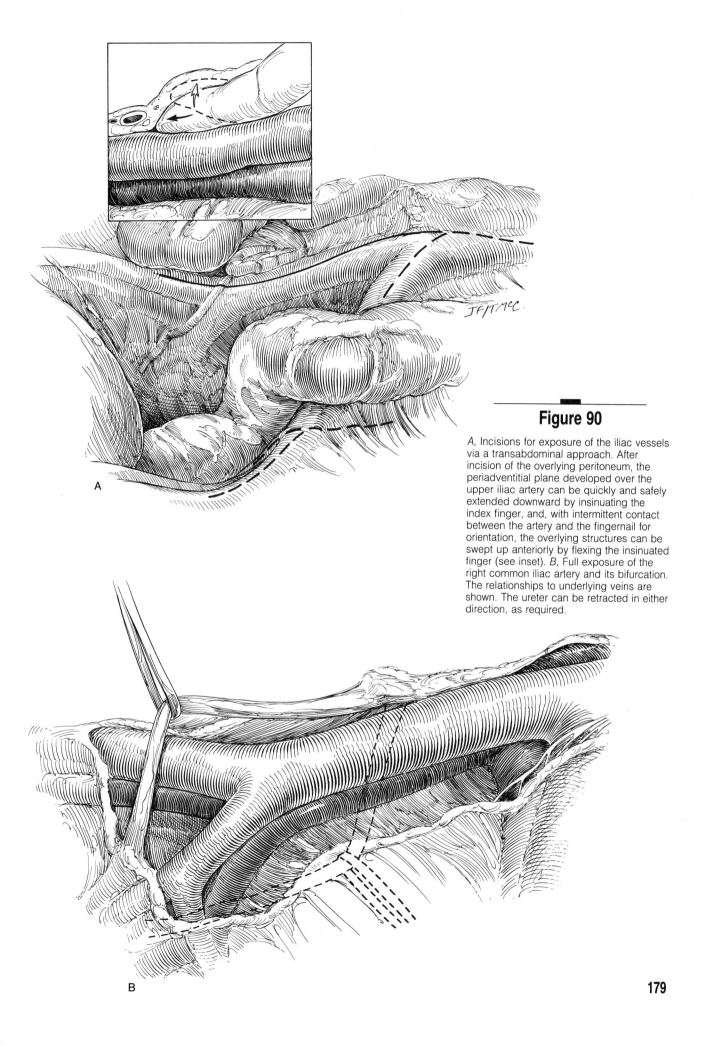

Figure 90

A, Incisions for exposure of the iliac vessels via a transabdominal approach. After incision of the overlying peritoneum, the periadventitial plane developed over the upper iliac artery can be quickly and safely extended downward by insinuating the index finger, and, with intermittent contact between the artery and the fingernail for orientation, the overlying structures can be swept up anteriorly by flexing the insinuated finger (see inset). *B,* Full exposure of the right common iliac artery and its bifurcation. The relationships to underlying veins are shown. The ureter can be retracted in either direction, as required.

A

B

Vascular Exposures

On the right side, the right iliac vein lies lateral to the right common iliac artery at first, but it progressively passes posterior to it as it gradually moves toward a completely medial position relative to the artery by the time it passes under the inguinal ligament. However, the proximal *right* iliac artery lies directly on top of the *left* iliac vein just beyond the aortic bifurcation and this is a notorious site of major iatrogenic venous injury. Dissection in the plane between the two vessels should be avoided whenever possible because they are often quite adherent and difficult to separate at this point, so much so that repair of the vein may require division of the artery. Of course, this is also the site of the "syndrome" left iliac vein compression. Beyond this dangerous crossroads, the left iliac vein progressively approaches the *left* common iliac artery and courses medial and deep to it and is less likely to be injured during this part of its course.

Knowing this anatomy, one should find it relatively easy to avoid common or external iliac vein injury when approaching the iliac artery bifurcations. However, the internal iliac (or hypogastric) veins lie close behind the arteries of the same name and must be carefully avoided in gaining exposure of the bifurcation of the iliac arteries. This is particularly true when dealing with aneurysmal disease, which is the most common situation when these vessels need to be dissected free, as opposed to occlusive disease wherein one usually bypasses the iliac bifurcations and tunnels down to the femoral arteries. Unless one finds very little inflammatory reaction around these vessels and/or adherence between them in this location, the safest approach to mobilizing the iliac bifurcation is shown sequentially in Figure 91*B* through *F*. The safest arterial segment to mobilize first is the external iliac artery. It often buckles upward just beyond its origin and is easily freed from the underlying vein. With an umbilical tape around it for traction, dissection proceeds upward past the bifurcation to the *common* iliac artery. With this traction helping to distract it from the underlying vein, an opening can usually be readily made between the common iliac artery and vein and a second umbilical tape inserted there. Then, with upward and inward (medial) traction on both, the hypogastric artery may be distracted from the underlying vein, enough for the former to be encircled with a tape (Fig. 91*A*). However, this last, most difficult maneuver is easily performed only in the minority of instances.

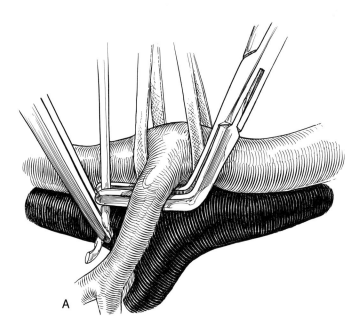

A

Figure 91

Encircling the hypogastric artery may occasionally be easily performed after traction is applied to the common and external iliac arteries *(A)*, but close application of the adjacent vein and inflammatory reaction and dense surrounding connective tissue often make this maneuver treacherous.

A safer approach to gaining control of the hypogastric artery is carried out by a maneuver often called (for no logical reason) "encirclement by subtraction." In actual practice, one progressively *adds* to the encirclement with an umbilical or a Silastic tape until a Potts double loop is completed. Ignoring the hypogastric artery itself, one first passes a tape inside-out under the external iliac artery below (Fig. 91*B*), then outside-in under the common iliac artery above (Fig. 91*C*), using the same openings developed when placing the other two umbilical tapes. This way all three elements of the iliac bifurcation are encircled. Then, if one wishes to *control* the hypogastric artery, the foregoing sequence is repeated once more in the same direction, as shown in Figure 91*D* and *E,* achieving control by the cinching action of a double (Potts) loop (Fig. 91*F*). For the sake of visual simplicity, the very tissues that make dissection difficult and this maneuver necessary are not apparent in these illustrations. This series of maneuvers can be used to advantage at other bifurcations and major branchings, most commonly in achieving control of the femoral bifurcation, with progressive encirclement of the profunda femoris artery as the final maneuver.

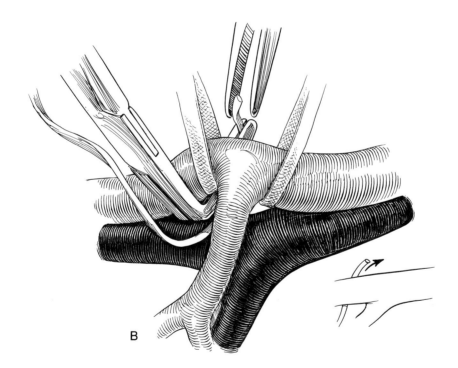

Figure 91 *Continued*

As described in the text, a safer alternative consists of first applying traction by tapes placed above and below the bifurcation and then encircling the hypogastric artery "by subtraction" *(B through F).*

Vascular Exposures

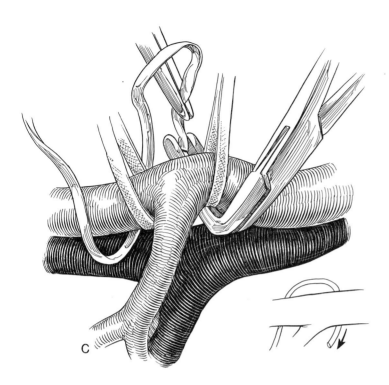

C

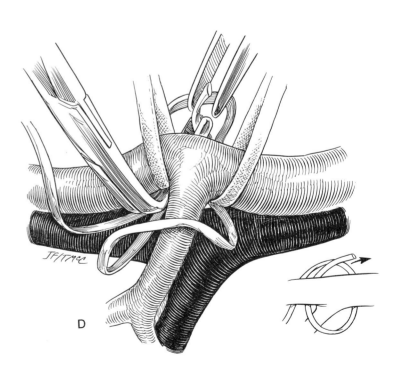

D

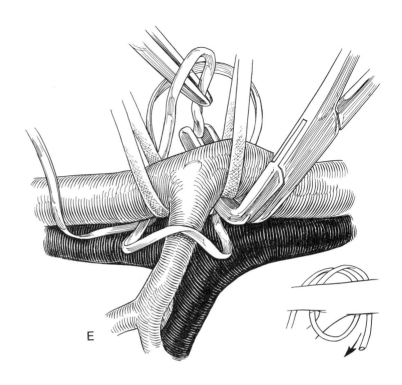

E

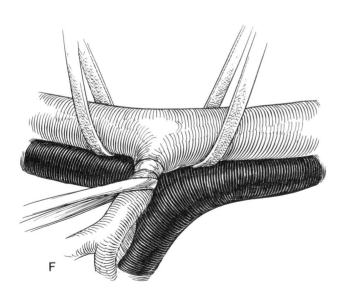

F

Vascular Exposures

Extraperitoneal Exposure of the Iliac Arteries. If one only needs to expose just the iliac arteries on one side, as in iliofemoral bypass or endarterectomy, it is not necessary, or even desirable, to open the abdomen widely. The iliac bifurcation may be adequately exposed through an extraperitoneal approach using the slightly oblique lower quadrant abdominal incision shown in Figure 92A. Even though originally borrowed from vascular surgery by transplant surgeons, this approach has come to be called the "renal transplant incision" because of its common use in this operation. Depending on whether the proximal common iliac artery or its bifurcation is the main focus of interest, the incision may be started at 1 to 2 FB above the midway point between the umbilicus and pubis, and be carried from the edge of the rectus muscle obliquely upward to a point 1 to 2 FB above and medial to the anterior superior iliac spine. After dividing or separating the external and internal oblique and transversus abdominalis muscles in line with this incision, the extraperitoneal plane is entered and bluntly developed superiorly and inferiorly before proceeding progressively around the peritoneal sac, retracting it medially and moving into the posterior extraperitoneal or "retroperitoneal" plane (Fig. 92B). With appropriately placed retractors, the iliac bifurcation is readily exposed (Fig. 92C). Its mobilization and control then proceed as described in the preceding section.

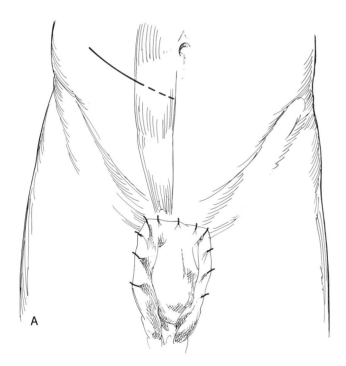

A

Figure 92

A, The incision for retroperitoneal exposure of the right iliac artery bifurcation. *B,* After dividing the abdominal muscles in line with the incision, the peritoneal sac and its contents are bluntly mobilized and then retracted upward and medially. *C,* The exposure of the right iliac bifurcation and the overlying ureter that is obtained through this incision.

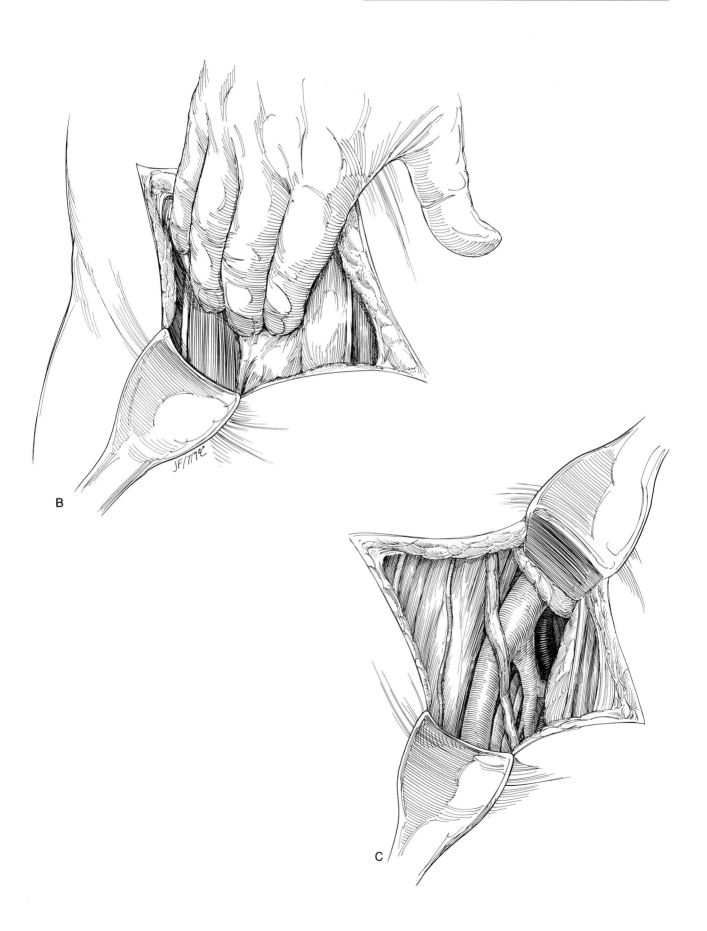

B

C

Vascular Exposures

Higher exposure, up to the aortoiliac junction, is easily obtained by moving this same retroperitoneal approach progressively upward an additional couple of fingerbreadths to provide exposure of the aortoiliac junction on one side and the same distance again to provide exposure for lumbar sympathectomy. The latter incision starts level with the umbilicus and ends laterally midway between the iliac crest and the lower costal margin (i.e., tip of the 12th rib). This or a slightly higher extraperitoneal approach on the right is adequate for caval ligation, clipping, or thrombectomy. On the left it may be used for aortic ligation in aneurysm exclusion and bypass.

Although exposure of the proximal common iliac artery is considerably shallower than exposure of the iliac bifurcation, it is also a site of predilection for arteriosclerotic plaquing and narrowing, and it carries a greater risk of injury to the underlying veins and, on the left side, of injury to the sympathetics coursing over the first part of the left common iliac artery. Therefore, when choosing a site for placing an anastomosis, exposure of the iliac bifurcation is often preferred, even though it is deeper. Finally, in presenting the applications of this incision, it should be mentioned that one can free up the extraperitoneal plane distally all the way down over the pelvic rim and, looking downward, proceed to expose the obturator foramen.

EXPOSURES OF THE SUPRARENAL AORTA

Proximal Control of the Aorta at the Diaphragm

In *emergency* situations when prompt proximal control of the aorta is required, the maneuver recommended by Veith may be lifesaving (Fig. 93A through D). The lesser omentum is opened vertically along the line shown in Figure 93A. Through this opening the crura are seen, and the left crus is bluntly split open in line with its fibers (Fig. 93B). Through this opening the index finger is inserted and, by sweeping away the loose areolar tissue around the aorta, superiorly and inferiorly and around both sides (Fig. 93C), the distal thoracic aorta is mobilized enough to accept a vascular clamp. This is best applied by inserting the index and middle fingers of one hand into the spaces developed on either side of the aorta and then guiding the tips of a large vascular clamp over them and into position. The clamp is closed when the tips "touch bottom"—that is, contact the thoracic spine and paraspinous muscles (Fig. 93D).

Exposure of the Suprarenal Aorta Using Medial Visceral Rotation

As stated earlier, significant suprarenal aortic exposure through a direct anterior approach requires medial visceral rotation, as popularized by Stoney. As shown in Figure 94A, this is performed by incising along the line of Toldt, first mobilizing the entire left colon (Fig. 94B), then the parietal attachments of the spleen (Fig. 94C). As the spleen is mobilized upward and medially, the tail of the pancreas is identified and mobilized medially with it. This carries one into a plane anterior to the left kidney and adrenal gland, which can be left in their beds.

Alternately, one can stay posteriorly and mobilize the kidney and adrenal gland forward, to expose the posterolateral aspect of the suprarenal aorta (Fig. 94*D*).

If one wishes to stay in front of the kidney and has difficulty finding the correct plane, one can enter this same plane lower down behind the colon and stay anterior to the ureter in approaching the infrarenal aorta. The latter is easily exposed, and one can then follow the anterior surface of the aorta up to the left renal vein. This plane anterior to the left kidney can be further developed upward to connect with the same plane achieved with mobilization of the spleen and pancreas to the right. Following this, the stomach can also be mobilized medially without dividing the short gastrics and, if advantageous, one can cut the diaphragmatic attachments of the left lobe of the liver and retract it to the right as well (the Grey-Turner maneuver). This gives full exposure of the aorta from the left crus of the diaphragm down (Fig. 94*E*). Then the crus itself can be divided to offer ready exposure of the supraceliac (lower thoracic) aorta (see inset of Fig. 94*E*) for proximal control or placement of the proximal anastomosis in an antegrade bypass to the celiac and/or superior mesenteric arteries.

Occlusion of the first part of the superior mesenteric artery may also be dealt with, through this approach although without much, if any, medial rotation of the spleen and pancreas, by "transposition" of the patent distal end of this artery to a convenient site on the aorta, usually just below the left renal vein. This same, more limited medial visceral rotation is also helpful in obtaining proximal aortic control when reoperating for failures of previous infrarenal aortic grafts (e.g., infection, occlusion, and aortoduodenal fistula). By this means one can gain suprarenal control of the aorta through normal tissue planes before approaching these difficult graft complications.

Direct Abdominal Versus Retroperitoneal Exposure of the Pararenal or Suprarenal Aorta. If the kidney and adrenal gland are left in place, as shown in Figure 94*E*, longitudinal aortic exposure is limited by the overlying left renal vein. Dissection of the periaortic tissue to the left of the superior mesenteric and celiac artery origins is often tedious because of numerous lymphatics, autonomic nerves, and small blood vessels. Thus, while antegrade mesenteric artery bypasses and endarterectomies of the visceral branches of the aorta are readily carried out with this exposure, bringing the kidney and adrenal gland forward with complete medial visceral rotation offers better exposure for suprarenal aneurysm repairs. The resultant exposure is shown in Figure 94*F*. However, when this maneuver is carried out through a direct transabdominal approach with the patient supine, the approach to the lateral or posterolateral aspect of the aorta can be a little awkward even if the surgeon stands to the patient's left and the operating table is tilted. Thus, if extensive suprarenal access is known to be required beforehand, the author prefers a left retroperitoneal approach (compare Fig. 94*F* with Fig. 104). If this need is realized intraoperatively, if full access to the right kidney or right iliac artery is also required, or if the abdominal contents must be carefully inspected afterwards, as in some mesenteric revascularizations, the direct abdominal approach with medial visceral rotation is chosen.

The vascular surgeon should be comfortable with the various modifications of both approaches and select the most appropriate one for the particular situation at hand. For example, left colon disease (diverticulitis, colon resection, or colostomy), retroperitoneal fibrosis (spontaneous or after irradiation), or certain caval or renal vein anomalies (left-sided cava, caval duplication) may mitigate against a *left* retroperitoneal approach, whereas this approach may be particularly

Vascular Exposures

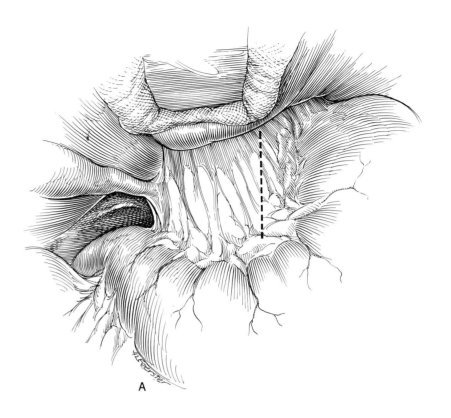

A

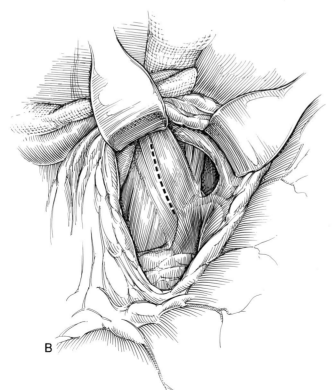

B

Figure 93

Sequential maneuvers for rapid exposure of the supraceliac aorta. *A,* Longitudinal opening in the lesser omentum. *B,* Blunt opening of the left crural fibers. *C,* Finger freeing the aorta from surrounding loose areolar tissue. *D,* Guiding the occluding vascular clamp in over two fingers until its tips "touch bottom" on the vertebral body behind the aorta.

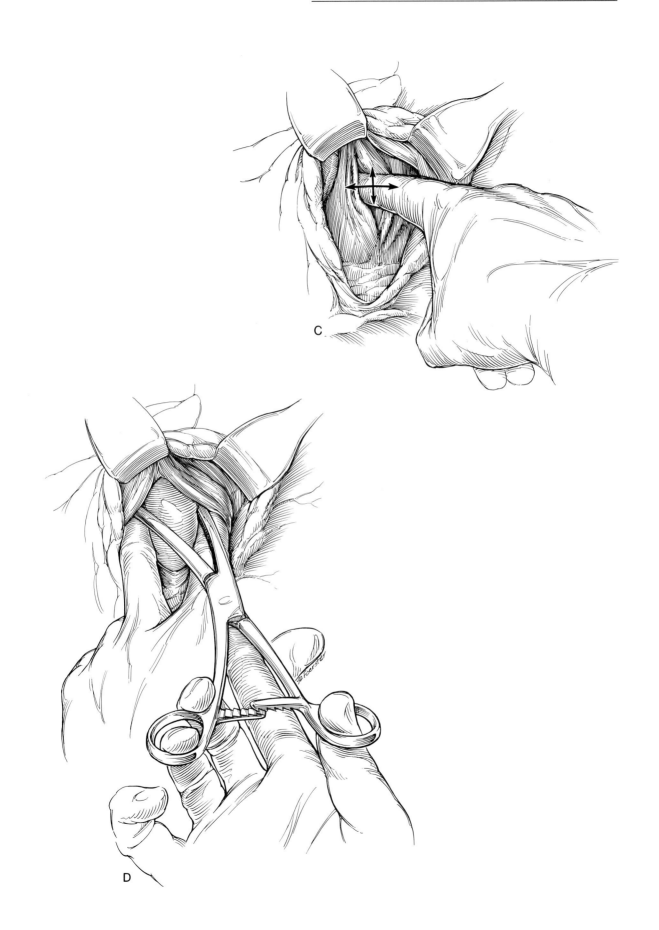

Vascular Exposures

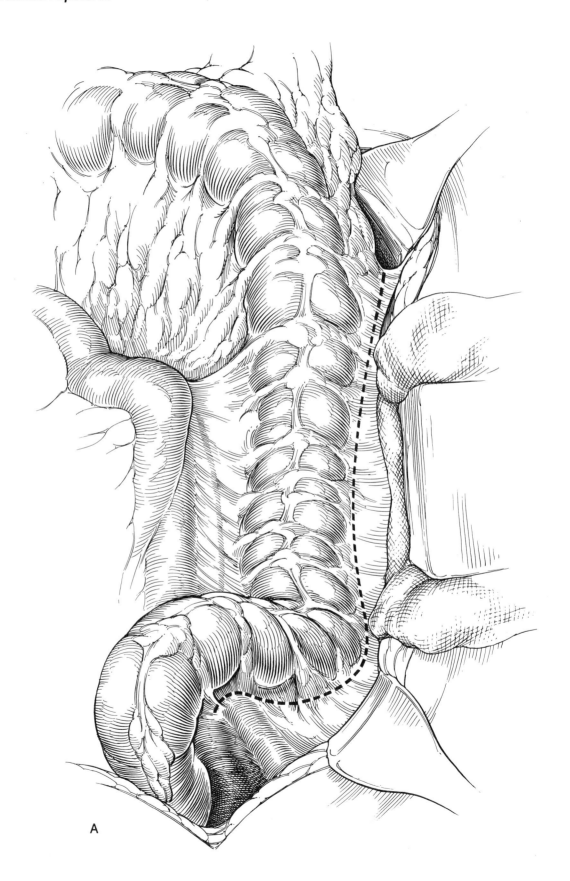

A

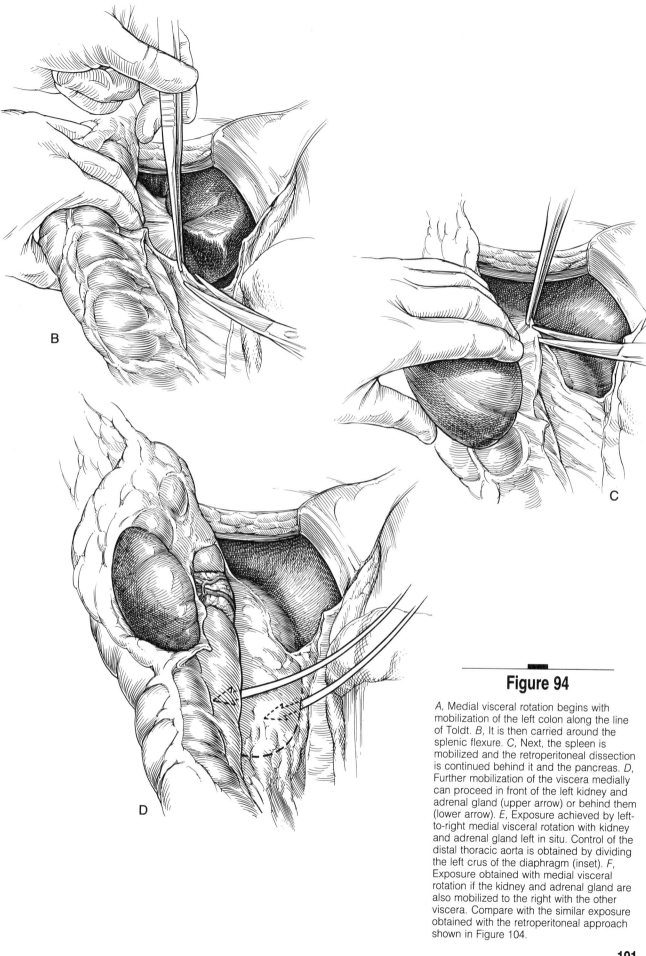

B

C

D

Figure 94

A, Medial visceral rotation begins with
mobilization of the left colon along the line
of Toldt. *B,* It is then carried around the
splenic flexure. *C,* Next, the spleen is
mobilized and the retroperitoneal dissection
is continued behind it and the pancreas. *D,*
Further mobilization of the viscera medially
can proceed in front of the left kidney and
adrenal gland (upper arrow) or behind them
(lower arrow). *E,* Exposure achieved by left-
to-right medial visceral rotation with kidney
and adrenal gland left in situ. Control of the
distal thoracic aorta is obtained by dividing
the left crus of the diaphragm (inset). *F,*
Exposure obtained with medial visceral
rotation if the kidney and adrenal gland are
also mobilized to the right with the other
viscera. Compare with the similar exposure
obtained with the retroperitoneal approach
shown in Figure 104.

Vascular Exposures

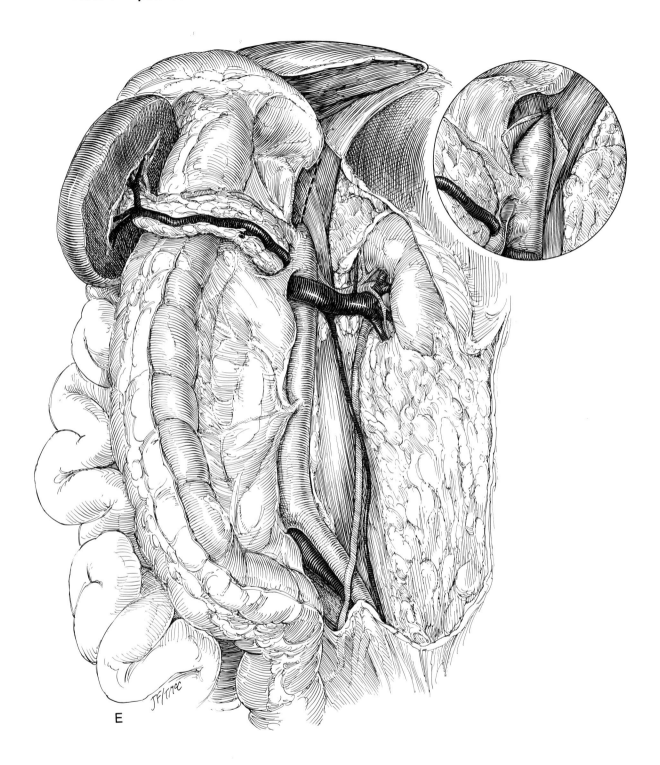

E

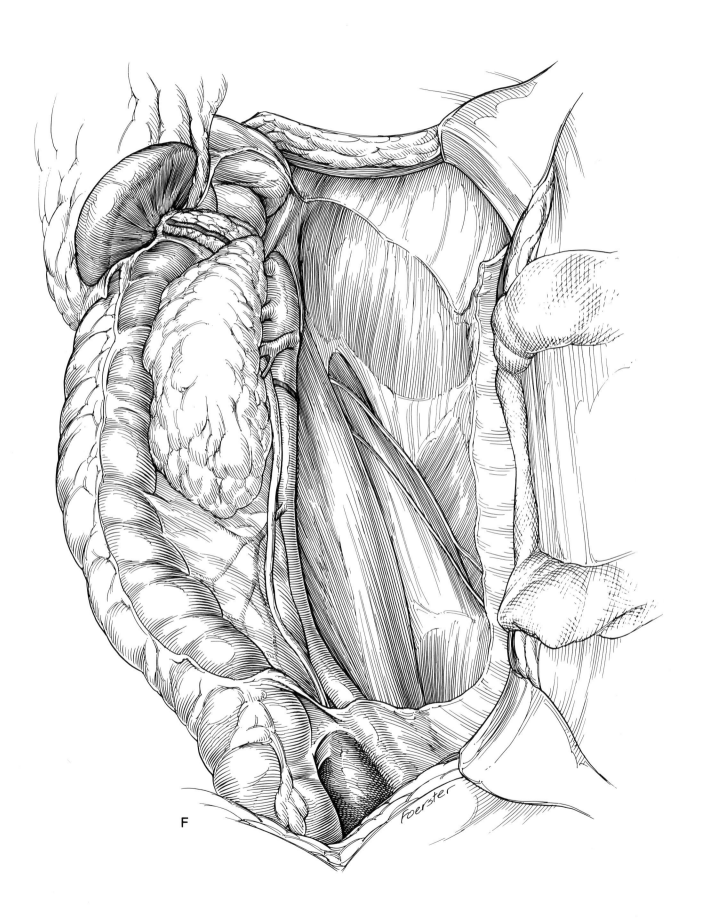

F

Vascular Exposures

helpful for the morbidly obese, for patients with severe pulmonary disease, for patients with previous abdominal operations with multiple adhesions, and for patients with aneurysms that are inflammatory or associated with horseshoe kidney. Through either approach, an associated retroaortic left renal vein can be more safely accommodated by leaving the kidney in situ.

Although specific reasons for choosing or avoiding the retroperitoneal approach have been given, debate continues over whether this approach has any generic advantages over transabdominal repair. A retrospective comparison between the two approaches carried out at Washington University School of Medicine in Saint Louis, Missouri, claimed certain advantages for the retroperitoneal approach (e.g., significantly less ileus and pulmonary complications and less time in the intensive care unit). A subsequent prospective trial at the Massachusetts General Hospital in Boston could *not* show statistically significant differences in these or other respects (although some mean values did favor the retroperitoneal approach). Because significant differences, similar to those of the Saint Louis study, *were* found when retrospective comparison was made with their own historical controls, the Boston group believed that advances in perioperative care rather than intrinsic differences were more responsible for the claimed advantages of the retroperitoneal approach. Nevertheless, this approach has gained increasing utilization, particularly among those graduating from institutions with vascular fellowships where it is widely utilized. The author prefers it, under the circumstances already mentioned for infrarenal aortic exposure, and prefers it even more for suprarenal aortic exposure, especially in operations performed for aneurysmal disease.

Retroperitoneal Approaches to the Abdominal Aorta

Difficulties may be encountered with the retroperitoneal approach if one tries to use only a single level of approach for all cases. As shown in Figure 95, one can use incisions keyed on the 12th, 11th, and 10th ribs. However, the body positioning differs between the upper and lower exposures. The lower of these incisions, from the tip of the 12th rib over to the midline or turned downward along the edge of the rectus muscle (Fig. 96A), requires the patient to be positioned on the right side with the table flexed at the level of the lumbar spine between the costal margins of the iliac crest (Fig. 96B). The chest and shoulders are elevated 45° to 60° from horizontal. The torso is twisted back to allow the hips to lie as close to horizontal as possible or with, at the most, 10° to 20° elevation (Fig. 96C). A deflatable "bean bag," in which irregularly shaped plastic pieces lock in position when the air is evacuated, provides firm, body-hugging contoured support and is ideal for holding this position and allowing the table to be rotated on its long axis to further adjust the position without body shifting. This allows the hips and pelvis to be tilted back later to the horizontal plane, permitting access to both groins if needed.

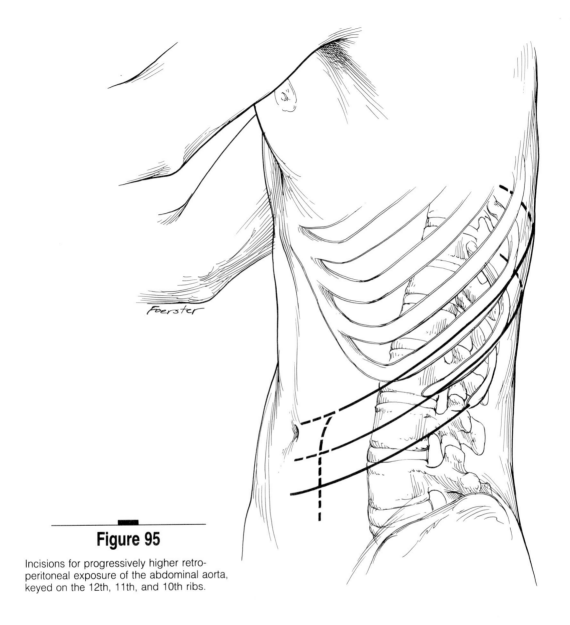

Figure 95

Incisions for progressively higher retroperitoneal exposure of the abdominal aorta,
keyed on the 12th, 11th, and 10th ribs.

Vascular Exposures

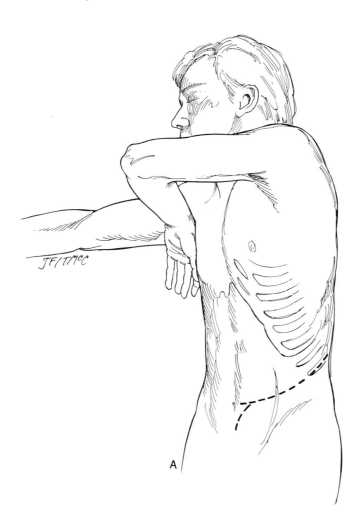

JF/TM°C

A

■

Figure 96

A, Incision for retroperitoneal exposure of the *infrarenal* aorta. *B and C,* Body positioning for this incision with upper torso at 45° and pelvis almost level.

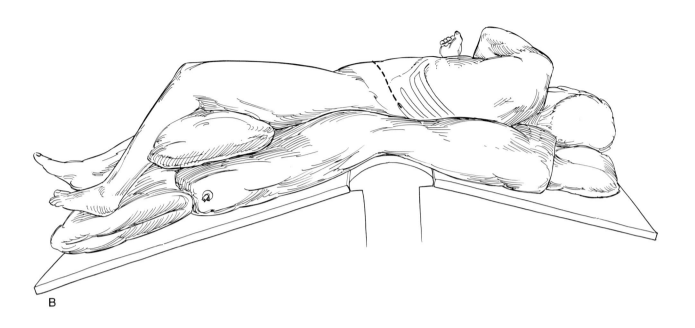

B

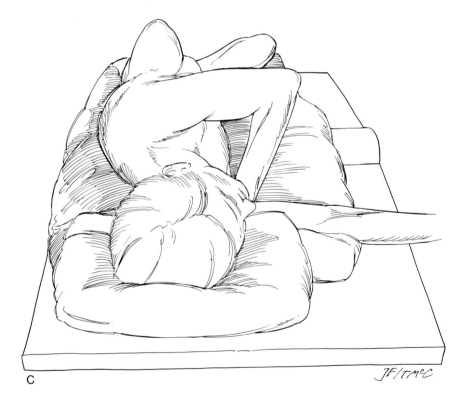

C

JF/TMcC

Vascular Exposures

After the incision is made and the underlying muscles are divided, the anterior edge of the properitoneal fat layer is encountered. At this time, a decision must be made whether the kidney is to be left down, in its bed, or whether it is to be mobilized up, with the abdominal contents (Fig. 97). Although the specific situations in which one or the other is preferred have already been discussed, the kidney is usually left *down* for *infrarenal* aortic exposures. If this is the case, one dissects *under* the properitoneal fat (arrow A, Fig. 98) and, by *widely* freeing up this retroperitoneal plane superiorly and inferiorly *before* proceeding posteriorly and mobilizing the peritoneal sac and its contents medially, one can ultimately achieve the exposure shown in Figure 99. It is best to approach the aorta first from below and then proceed upward, passing over the iliopsoas muscle and in front of the ureter and gonadal vessels to reach the distal aorta or upper left iliac artery. Following in that plane, dissect upward to the level of the left renal vein. The inferior mesenteric artery will be encountered, but on the opposite side of the field than one is used to with the direct transabdominal approach. If patent, it must be preserved and protected. This approach is useful for repair of infrarenal aortic aneurysms without major involvement of the right iliac artery.

If, on the other hand, the kidney is to be mobilized upward with the other viscera, one stays *behind* the properitoneal fat and Gerota's fascia initially (arrow B, Fig. 98). By mobilizing the kidney up, the left renal vein is no longer an impediment to higher exposure. Furthermore, with the kidney and adrenal gland moved forward, the lateral aspect of the suprarenal aorta can be approached, once the descending lumbar vein is divided. The resulting exposure (Fig. 100) is ideal for juxtarenal or pararenal involvement.

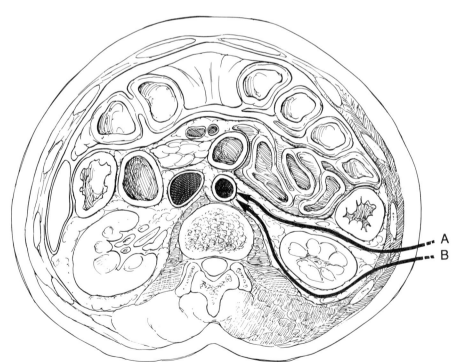

A
B

Figure 97

Two approaches into the retroperitoneal structures—one anterior to the kidney and adrenal gland *(A)*; the other behind these organs, mobilizing them forward *(B)*.

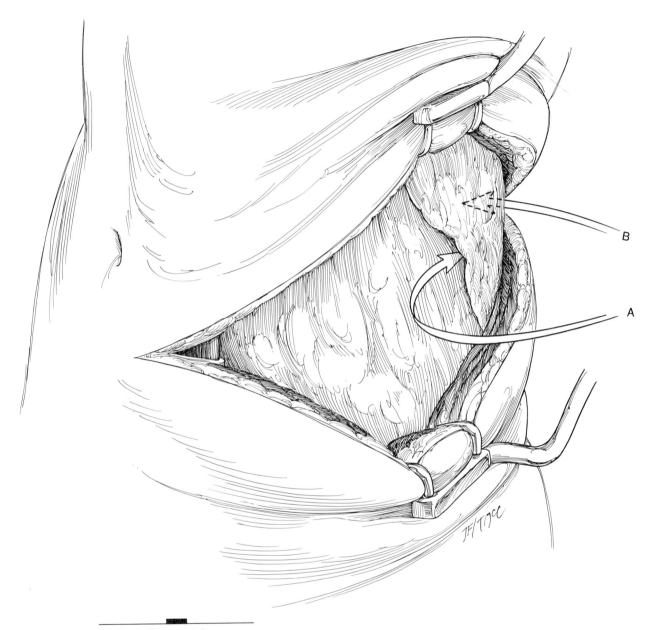

Figure 98

Depending on the approach selected, one proceeds in front of the preperitoneal fat pad, which is contiguous with Gerota's fascia, and in front of the kidney (A), or one proceeds outside of the fat pad and behind the kidney (B).

Vascular Exposures

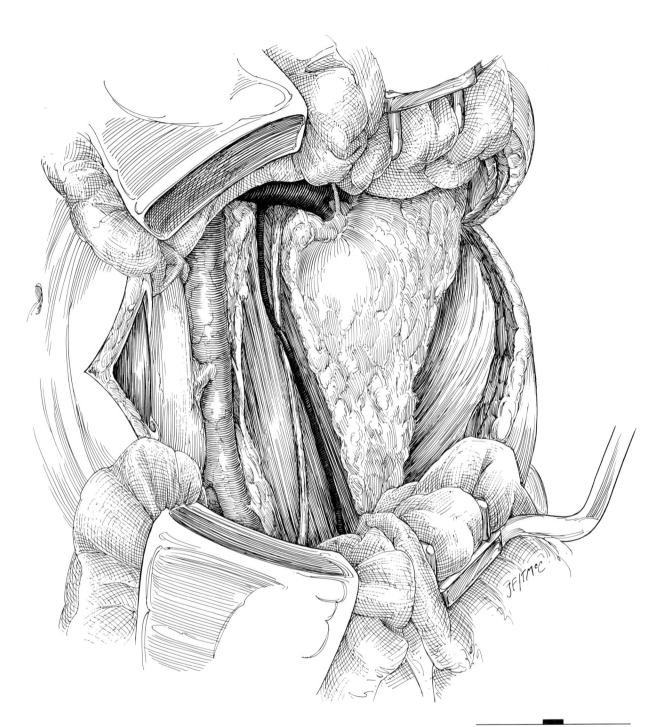

Figure 99

The aortic exposure obtained through the 12th-rib retroperitoneal approach when the kidney is left in situ is adequate for most infrarenal procedures.

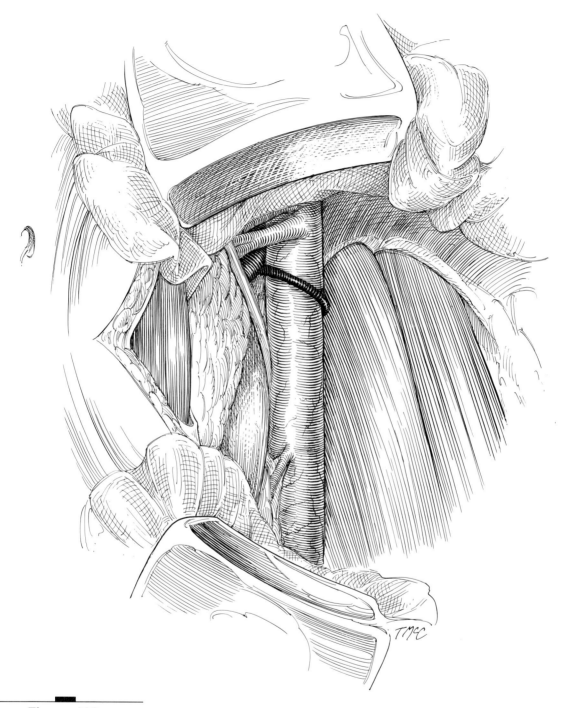

Figure 100

The aortic exposure obtained through the
12th-rib retroperitoneal approach when the
left kidney and adrenal gland are mobilized
upward and medially is suitable for dealing
with juxtarenal involvement.

Vascular Exposures

For higher exposure one can move up to the level of the 11th or even 10th rib with the incision being carried back to the paraspinous muscles to allow full rib excision (Fig. 101A). With these higher exposures, the patient's upper torso must be positioned farther forward so that the shoulders are *perpendicular* to the operating table, and the pelvis, after the trunk is twisted and flexed, is lying at 30° (Fig. 101B). Again, using the bean bag, the patient can be rotated on the long axis in this position so that the shoulders drop back to 60° and the pelvis is almost horizontal, but it is better to start with the higher position. As Mel Williams, who popularized this approach, has warned, high exposure can easily be obtained *only* with the upper torso in a full lateral (90°) position.

Whether one goes between ribs or through the bed of a resected rib is a matter of personal preference. Through the bed gives slightly wider exposure and is less likely to break a rib or injure an intercostal nerve, in the author's opinion. Rib removal causes no more incisional discomfort. However, significant incisional pain and/or denervation bulging of the flank should be anticipated in about 10% of patients with these incisions. Figure 102A and B shows subperiosteal removal of the 11th rib. The tip of the pleura is found directly under this rib, with its telltale glistening white surface. It can be avoided by carefully dissecting under its sharp, sloping inferior edge and mobilizing it upward (Fig. 102C). Once that is accomplished, the anterior half of the incision is deepened, much as that for the previously described incision at the 12th rib level, down to the properitoneal fat. The tip of the rib is the most reliable point of entrance into this plane; furthermore, it is easier and safer to mobilize the properitoneal superiorly and inferiorly if one proceeds from lateral to medial rather than the reverse. Again, the choice between going in front of or behind the kidney is determined in advance, and by entering in front of or behind the properitoneal fat layer, one can initiate these different exposures. Staying anterior to the kidney is ideal for renal artery reconstruction, particularly aortorenal bypass, and for mesenteric revascularizations. This exposure is seen in Figure 103.

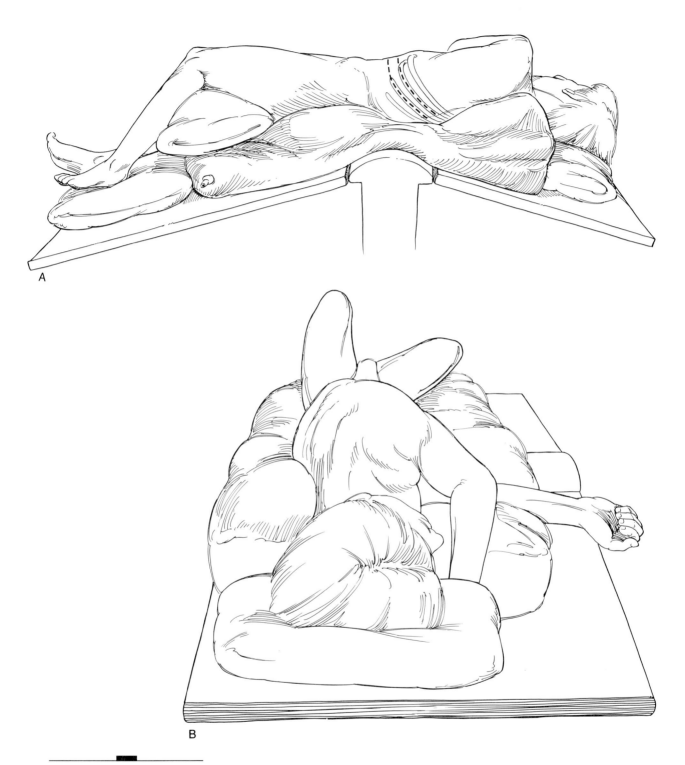

A

B

Figure 101

A and B, Body position for higher (10th- and 11th-rib) retroperitoneal approaches; upper torso at 90° and pelvis at 30°. Use of beanbag holds position and allows axial tilt adjustments to suit different stages of the operation.

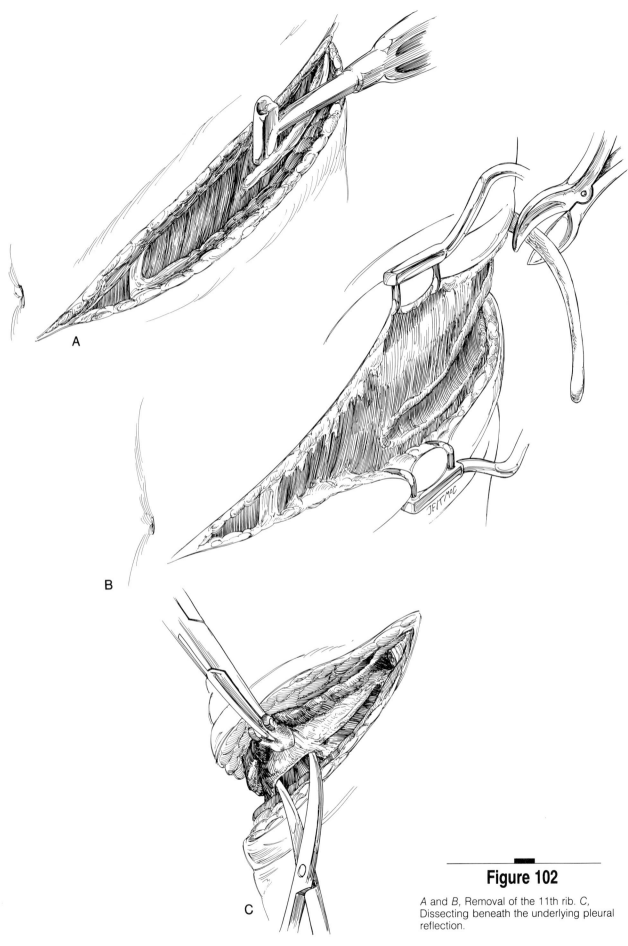

Figure 102

A and *B*, Removal of the 11th rib. *C*,
Dissecting beneath the underlying pleural
reflection.

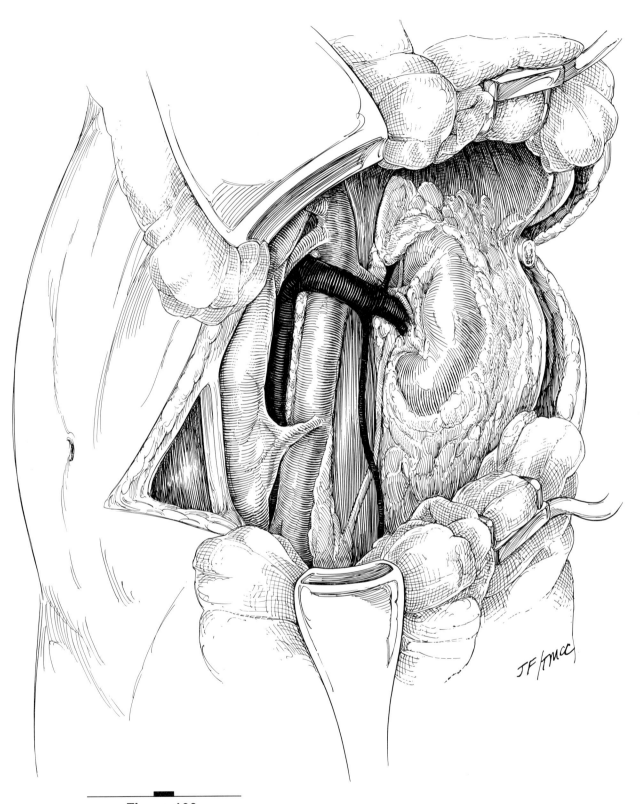

Figure 103

Exposure obtained with the kidney and
adrenal gland left in situ.

Vascular Exposures

Staying behind the kidney and adrenal gland gives higher exposure and, if the 10th rib or interspace is chosen, one can obtain excellent exposure of the entire suprarenal abdominal aorta and obtain proximal control of the distal thoracic aorta by opening the left crus of the diaphragm. One almost invariably enters the pleura with the 10th-rib approach. This can be easily repaired and the pleura evacuated at the time of closure. On other occasions, the posterior rim of the diaphragm can be deliberately detached, allowing wider exposure of the lower thoracic aorta. The usual exposure obtained through the 11th rib incision is seen in Figure 104. Particularly with aneurysmal disease, control of the aorta just above the diaphragm is preferable to attempting to dissect around the aorta lower down because of denser periaortic tissues containing lymphatics and autonomic nerves that lie along the anterior surfaces near the origins of the celiac and superior mesenteric arteries. For the foregoing reasons, the author prefers the 11th rib approach for exposure anterior to the kidney and the 10th rib approach for higher exposure, staying posterior to the kidney.

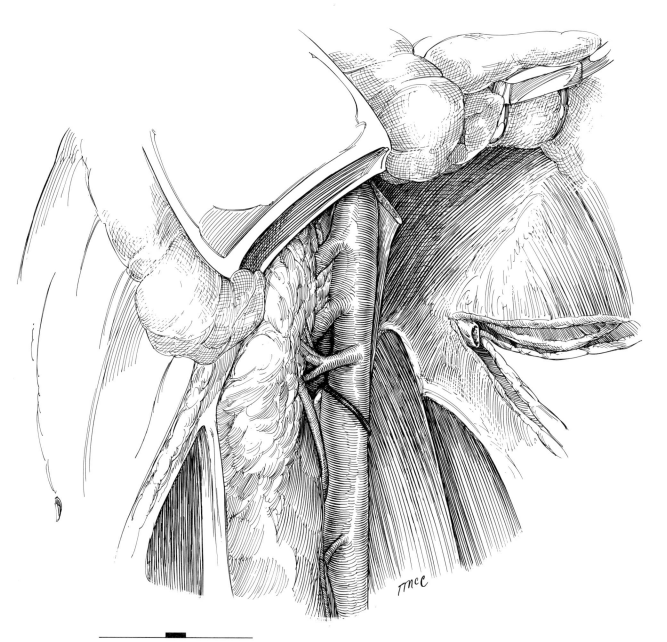

Figure 104

Exposure obtained with the kidney and
adrenal gland mobilized and retracted
medially.

Vascular Exposures

The Risberg Incision. One disadvantage of left retroperitoneal approaches through transverse or oblique incisions is that, if the incision is placed high, it is difficult to reach the aortic bifurcation and the upper iliac arteries (especially the right), whereas if it is placed low, the upper levels of the suprarenal aorta are not easily reachable. When one needs exposure from the upper abdominal aorta to the iliacs, one solution is a long midline incision with medial visceral rotation. However, in those specific circumstances in which the left retroperitoneal approach offers definite advantages over direct transabdominal exposure, another option has been suggested by the Swedish surgeon Risberg. As shown in Figure 105, the incision is made just lateral to the rectus sheath in a semilunar line which is carried right up to the costal margin. However, the costal margin is not normally divided, rather the muscles *under* it are separated away and divided to allow the underlying peritoneum to be exposed. The properitoneal plane is developed, as in any other retroperitoneal approach, throughout the length of the incision until the abdominal viscera, enclosed in their peritoneal sac, can be retracted medially. The difference with this incision is that this is carried out through a longitudinal incision and therefore exposes a greater length of the abdominal aorta.

The upper part of the peritoneal dissection should be performed last because inadvertent entry into the peritoneum is more likely here. Once the incision has been carried down just lateral to the rectus sheath into the properitoneal plane, this plane should be developed on a broad front inferiorly and superiorly, taking advantage of the fact that the dissection is easier in the lower parts of the abdomen. Only after the dissection plane has been well established and completed inferiorly should one approach the upper aspect of the incision near the costal margin. After extensive mobilization of the peritoneal sac, this incision gives good exposure from well above the renal arteries to below the aortic bifurcation. It produces no more discomfort or denervation than that of the transverse extraperitoneal approaches, as only the left rectus muscle is likely to be affected by this dissection. The only relative disadvantages are difficulty staying out of the abdominal cavity superiorly and the extensiveness of the extraperitoneal dissection. For those familiar with extraperitoneal dissection, the latter is not a disadvantage. For most surgeons, however, use of this approach will be limited to those special circumstances when this longer exposure is required and one is dealing with "hostile" abdominal pathology, such as multiple adhesions, horseshoe kidneys, or inflammatory aneurysm, and one needs to use an extraperitoneal approach.

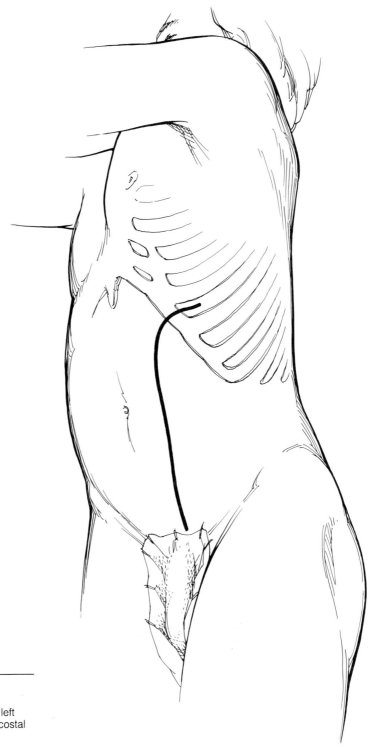

Figure 105

The Risberg incision, along the left semilunar line and up over the costal margin.

ALTERNATIVE EXPOSURES OF UPPER ABDOMINAL VISCERAL ARTERIES

Before leaving the abdomen and continuing on up into the thorax for even higher aortic exposures, it is appropriate to discuss alternative exposures of major visceral arteries in the upper abdomen. These can be carried out through right or left retroperitoneal incisions, or transabdominally through the incisions shown in Figure 106. Exposure of the renal hilus through an open abdomen can be achieved as an extension of aortic exposure when performed as an adjunct to aortic surgery; but, if the primary focus is renal revascularization, it is often easier to reflect the colon medially. Here either an upper midline or chevron incision is appropriate. However, for elective unilateral renal artery reconstructions, the author prefers the exposure offered by a left or right retroperitoneal approach through the 11th rib. This not only is well tolerated but also brings the anatomy closer and is far preferable to working in the depths of the abdomen, retracting loops of bowel out of the way.

On the *left* side of the abdomen, higher up, a number of vascular operations involving the splenic and renal vessels can be performed with basically similar exposures. For exposure of the splenic and left renal veins, either an extended upper midline or left chevron incision may be used. Transabdominally, if one wishes to stay *below* the transverse mesocolon, the small bowel is retracted to the right, the colon drawn upward over the abdomen, and the duodenum completely mobilized to the right (Fig. 107*A*). This exposes the inferior mesenteric vein, which leads up to the splenic vein, and the left renal vein (Fig. 107*B*). The pancreas determines the upper limits of this exposure. Alternatively, one can achieve this same exposure by going *above* the transverse colon, entering the omental sac through the avascular plane where the *undersurface* of the greater omentum joins the surface of the transverse colon. The deeper exposure begins with dissecting along the lower edge of the pancreas, under which lies the splenic vein, and subsequently moving down to the left renal vein (Fig. 108*A* and *B*). The latter is the usual approach for the most common splenorenal venous anastomosis, the Warren shunt. The final exposure is seen in Figure 108*C*.

If a splenic to renal *artery* anastomosis is intended, it is better to begin out at the splenic hilus, after mobilizing the colon medially. The splenic artery can be divided there, leaving the spleen supplied by the short gastrics. Then one can dissect out the splenic artery from that point down, steadily mobilizing the pancreas upward in the process. After achieving sufficient mobilization of this artery, one can then move downward to expose the left renal artery, which usually lies slightly superior and deep to the left renal vein. Some degree of medial visceral rotation is required here, whether the approach is transabdominal or completely extraperitoneal.

Exposure of the Superior Mesenteric Artery. In both the transabdominal (see Fig. 94) and retroperitoneal approaches (see Figs. 103 and 104) to the suprarenal aorta, the opportunities for exposure of the *origin* of the superior mesenteric artery have already been mentioned. If one stays in front of the kidney in either approach, the proximal segment of the superior mesenteric artery can be readily mobilized and, if there is a short occlusion, the artery can be transected and turned down for anastomosis into the aorta. This transposition of the artery is a relatively simple approach to chronic mesenteric ischemia in that it requires no graft and just a single anastomosis. The resulting aortomesenteric anastomosis usually ends up being positioned just above or below the left renal vein, to the right of the midline on the abdominal aorta. If exposure of both the celiac and superior mesenteric arteries is required, as well as the adjacent aorta, either the transabdominal approach with medial visceral rotation or the highest of the left retroperitoneal approaches serves well. A third option is to approach these vessels directly anteriorly, just below the aortic hiatus in the diaphragm. This is a more deliberate extension of the previously described approach to obtaining rapid control of the subdiaphragmatic aorta (see Fig. 93A through D). After dividing the left crus and getting proximal aortic control, a considerable amount of distal thoracic aorta can be mobilized along with the origins of the celiac and superior mesenteric arteries. With this exposure it is possible to perform a short bypass or limited endarterectomy, but it is not a favorite approach of the author.

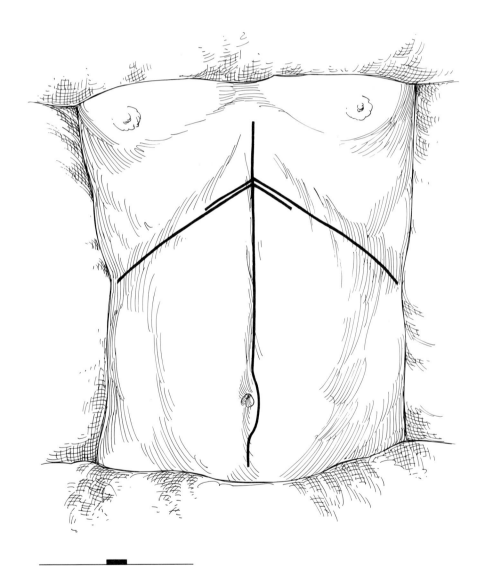

Figure 106

Incisions for transabdominal exposure of the major upper abdominal aortic or caval branches: midline and right or left subcostal chevron.

Vascular Exposures

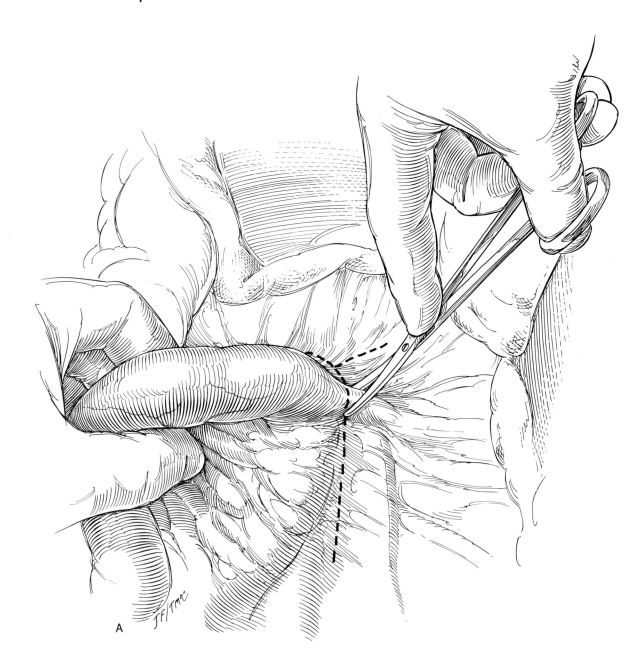

A

JF/TMcC

Figure 107

A, Mobilizing the duodenum at the ligament
of Treitz, to reach the splenorenal vessels.
B, After upward retraction on the edge of
the pancreas, the splenic, inferior
mesenteric, and left renal veins are seen, as
are the aorta and the left renal artery.

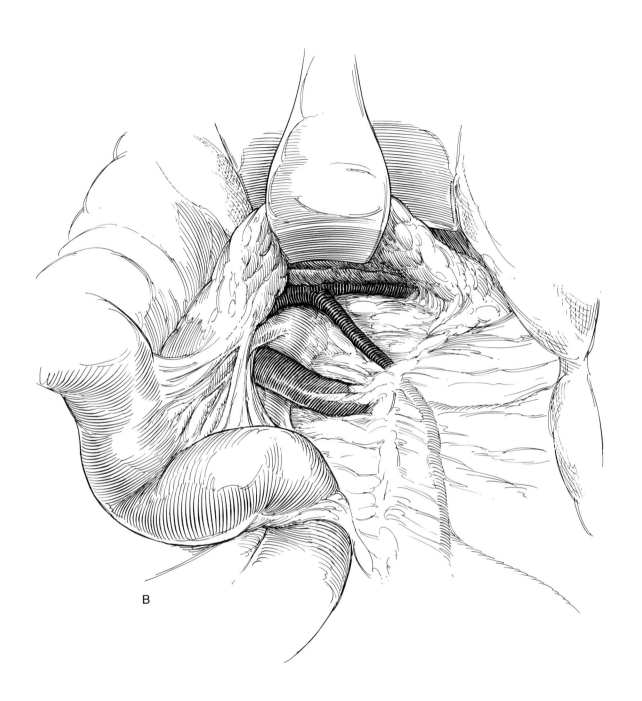

B

Vascular Exposures

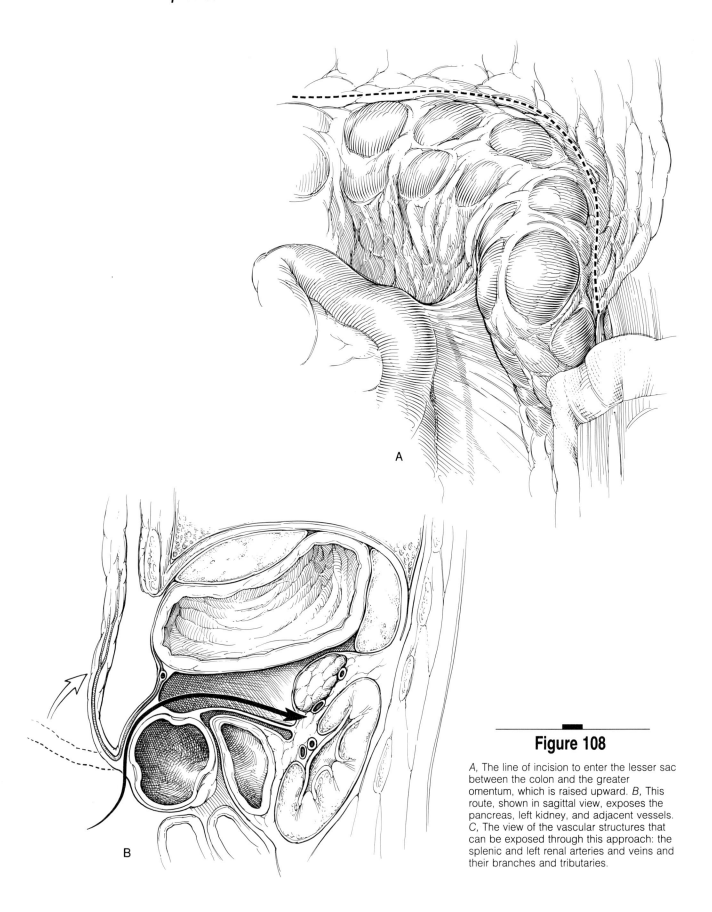

A

B

Figure 108

A, The line of incision to enter the lesser sac between the colon and the greater omentum, which is raised upward. *B,* This route, shown in sagittal view, exposes the pancreas, left kidney, and adjacent vessels. *C,* The view of the vascular structures that can be exposed through this approach: the splenic and left renal arteries and veins and their branches and tributaries.

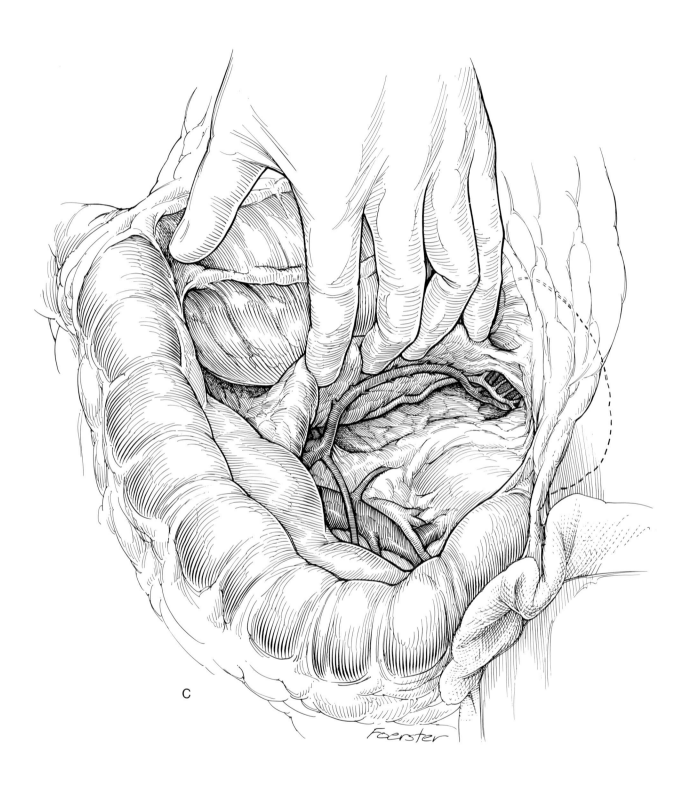

c

Foerster

Vascular Exposures

If one wishes to expose the more distal segment of the superior mesenteric artery through the base of the mesentery, as is commonly required in dealing with *acute* mesenteric ischemia and for performing retrograde aortomesenteric anastomoses, a long midline incision is made. The transverse colon is retracted superiorly and the base of the mesentery is grasped in the fingers (Fig. 109*A*). If the superior mesenteric artery is pulsatile, it can be felt easily between the thumb and index finger through the mesentery. Even in chronic occlusions, a hand-held Doppler probe will help localize the artery if it is patent distal to the occlusion. But this is *not* applicable in *acute* mesenteric ischemia. Palpation of the upper superior mesenteric in this manner may detect no proximal pulse (arterial thrombosis) or a proximal pulse that abruptly stops (mesenteric embolus). In the

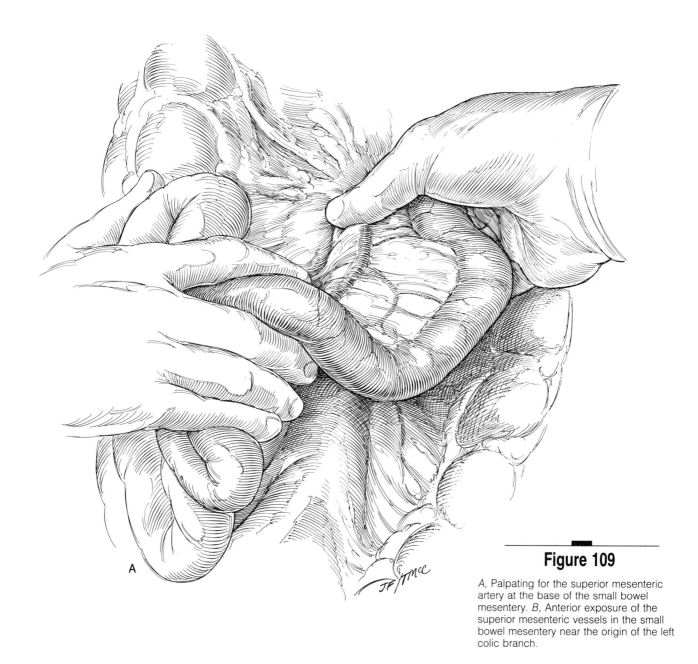

A

Figure 109

A, Palpating for the superior mesenteric artery at the base of the small bowel mesentery. *B,* Anterior exposure of the superior mesenteric vessels in the small bowel mesentery near the origin of the left colic branch.

latter circumstance, the upper jejunum will be viable; in the former, it will not be viable. In either event, the best approach here is to expose the superior mesenteric artery high in the mesentery on its anterolateral surface. Even if the artery is occluded and there is little or no distal flow detectable by Doppler interrogation, the probe can still detect flow in the superior mesenteric vein, which lies slightly behind and to the left of the artery. Even if there are no *spontaneous* sounds in the vein, one can detect a telltale rush when the mesentery is squeezed. A vertical incision made over these vessels usually exposes them near the origin of the middle colic artery. Most emboli lodge just at or beyond this. In thromboses, the entire segment may be occluded. Figure 109*B* shows the exposure of the segment of the superior mesenteric artery obtained by this approach.

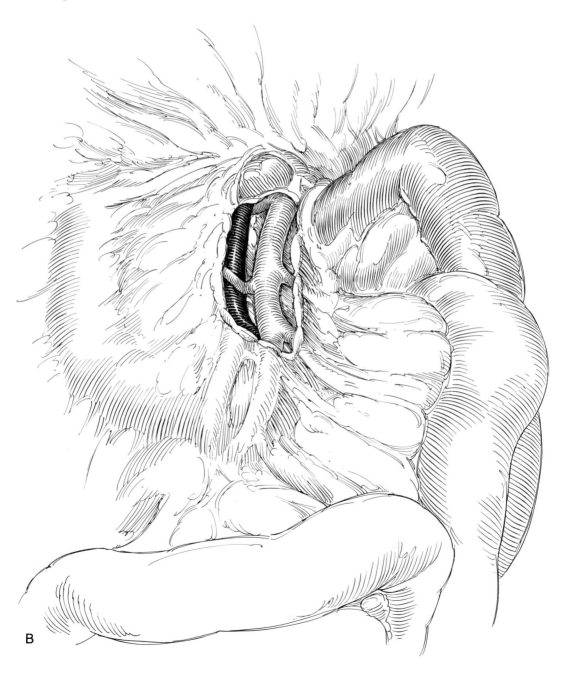

B

Vascular Exposures

Right-Sided Approaches to Abdominal Visceral Vessels. A right-sided retroperitoneal approach is appropriate for right renal artery revascularization and can be used to advantage to deal with an aortic aneurysm associated with a right iliac artery aneurysm, an aberrant right renal artery, a horseshoe kidney in which the arterial anatomy is best approached from the right, or an aneurysm associated with either a left-sided vena cava or vena caval transposition, to avoid direct confrontation with these large veins. All of these circumstances could be well managed through incisions that are essentially mirror images of those on the left already described (see Figs. 100, 103, and 104). They will not be illustrated again here. More limited right retroperitoneal approaches are appropriate for localized procedures on the inferior vena cava or a right lumbar sympathectomy. A mesocaval shunt requires a transabdominal approach, but this operation is rarely performed now. Most of the other operations requiring extensive exposure of the inferior vena cava, the left renal artery or vein, or the vascular structures in the porta hepatis can be approached through either a long upper midline or left chevron incision with mobilization of the colon and duodenum to the right. This is described.

The right colon is reflected to the left (Fig. 110*A*). This exposes the infrarenal vena cava and upper iliac veins and arteries (lower inset, Fig. 110*C*) and in some instances the renal veins, but higher exposure requires mobilization of the duodenum (Fig. 110*B*). Mobilization of the duodenum provides higher exposure of not only the suprarenal vena cava and both renal veins (Fig. 110*C*) but also the portal vein, which lies inferiorly, deep in the porta hepatis (upper inset, Fig. 110*C*). Through this exposure, the proper hepatic artery can also be exposed anteriorly in the porta hepatis where it usually lies slightly behind and to the right of the common bile duct. After it leaves the celiac axis, the common hepatic artery ultimately gives off a large gastroduodenal branch before becoming the proper hepatic artery and traveling up into the porta hepatis. As shown in the upper inset of Figure 110*C*, the junction of the gastroduodenal artery with the hepatic artery is important in performing a hepatorenal bypass. It is usually selected for the proximal anastomosis, and in some instances the gastroduodenal branch itself is large enough to serve this purpose. In others the arteriotomy can be extended into the origin of the gastroduodenal artery to provide a wider, beveled anastomosis. The aforementioned approach, with the described modifications, gives adequate exposure for almost all operations on visceral vessels lying to the right of the midline.

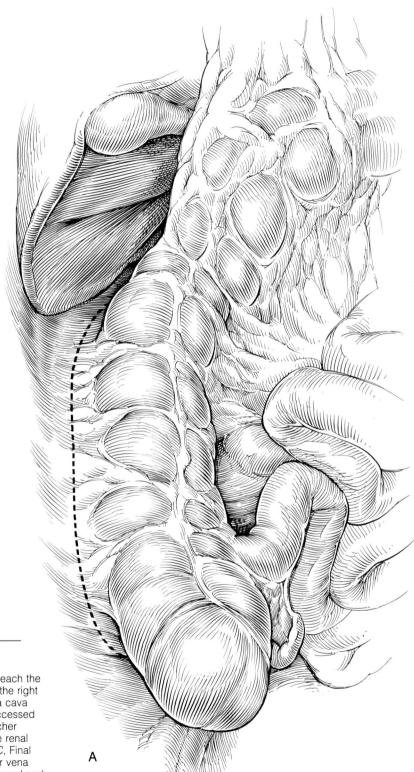

Figure 110

A, Reflection of the right colon to reach the major right-sided vessels. *B,* With the right colon reflected, the infrarenal vena cava and common iliac veins can be accessed but duodenal reflection by the Kocher maneuver additionally exposes the renal veins and suprarenal vena cava. *C,* Final exposure of the subhepatic inferior vena cava and its major tributaries, the renal and iliac veins (lower inset). By dissecting up into the porta hepatis from below (upper inset), the hepatic artery at the point of origin of its gastroduodenal branch can be exposed as needed for hepatorenal shunt.

A

Vascular Exposures

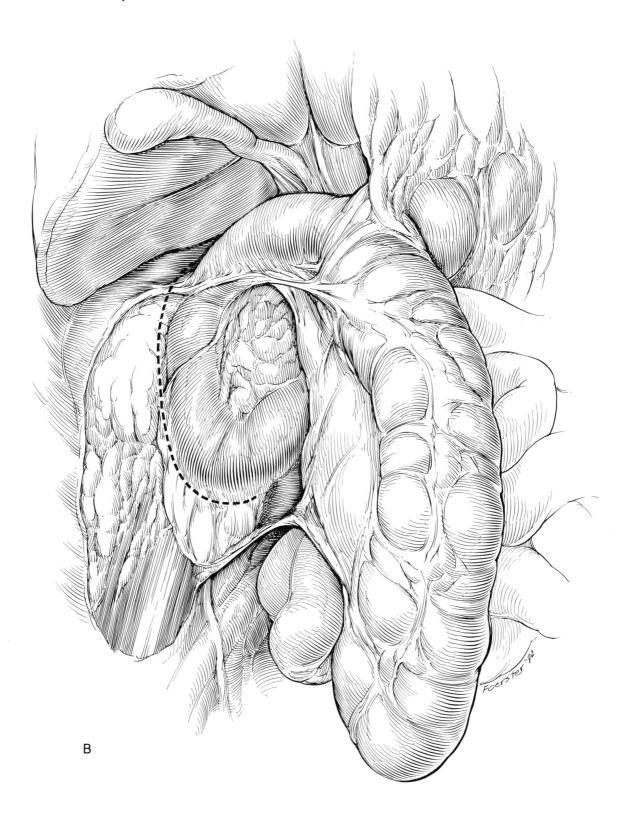

B

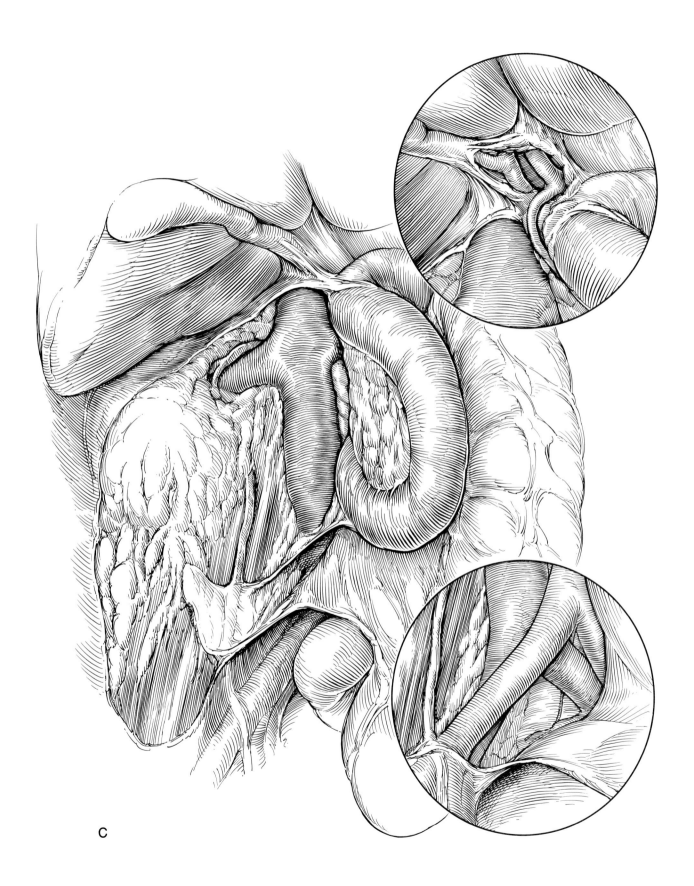

c

THORACOABDOMINAL AORTIC EXPOSURES

Operations on the thoracic aorta, performed through the exposures described subsequently, are no longer considered difficult technically, thanks to the innovative simplifications introduced by Stanley Crawford. The dissections and anastomoses do not rank with those of a difficult distal bypass, a complicated abdominal aortic aneurysm repair, or most reoperative vascular surgery. Like many cardiac procedures and proximal aortic surgery, it is "getting there and getting back safely" that is the challenge. High among these challenges are protection of the spinal cord and abdominal viscera against ischemia and avoidance of major hemodynamic changes when clamping and unclamping the aorta close to the heart. A certain freedom, however, is associated with operating through a wide open thoracotomy on such large, accessible arterial segments, usually without much overlying tissue, nearby veins, or adjacent nerves. Currently, with the remarkable progress made in anesthetic techniques, autotransfusion, perioperative monitoring, and intensive care, and with the promise held by studies into the prevention of paraplegia associated with thoracic aortic cross-clamping, it can be anticipated that thoracoabdominal aortic surgery will soon be much safer and more widely performed.

When operating on the thoracoabdominal aorta, the choice of incision depends largely on the extent of the disease. If the upper limit of disease is the lower descending thoracic aorta, an eighth interspace incision will suffice. But if the occluding clamp will be placed just below the left subclavian artery, the fifth or sixth interspace (or rib) should be chosen. The posterior limit of these thoracic incisions reaches to the paraspinous muscles and therefore it is always necessary to expose and prepare the skin right down to the spinous processes. If the distal extent of the disease ends at the renal arteries, the thoracotomy may need to be extended forward only to the edge of the rectus muscle. If exposure of the aortic bifurcation is needed, the incision must be turned down and carried into the lower abdomen. To stay extraperitoneally, it is best to stay just outside the edge of the rectus muscle and proceed down along the semilunar line. But this exposure will comfortably reach only to just below the renal arteries. For greater distal exposure, especially if the right iliac arteries need to be included in the field, the incision should be carried over to the midline and down its full length, with the abdomen opened widely and the viscera rotated medially. As shown in Figure 111, most of these incisions can be made with the patient in the same basic position. The right chest or the upper torso is elevated up to between 70° and 90° and the hips and pelvis are left as flat as possible (i.e., up only 10° to 20°), with the table slightly flexed at the level of the upper lumbar vertebrae. A right axillary roll is used for protection and a deflatable bean bag is used to hold the twisted torso in this position, keeping it from slipping back down toward the horizontal. Its firm contour-hugging feature also allows table rotation without body shifting.

The first thoracoabdominal exposure to be described here is actually a superior approach to the suprarenal and distal thoracic aorta, exposing much of the same anatomy one might reach through a high (10th rib) left retroperitoneal approach (see Figure 104), but here it is exposed through the chest via a lower (eighth to ninth interspace) left thoracotomy. This approach has the generic morbidity of a thoracotomy but usually provides somewhat better exposure, without the need for much dissection or strong retraction. Thus it may be preferred in those patients whose pulmonary status does not constitute a contraindication (for thoracotomy) and in whom one wishes to perform an endarterectomy for occlusive disease of the upper abdominal aorta or to repair aneurysmal disease, primarily involving

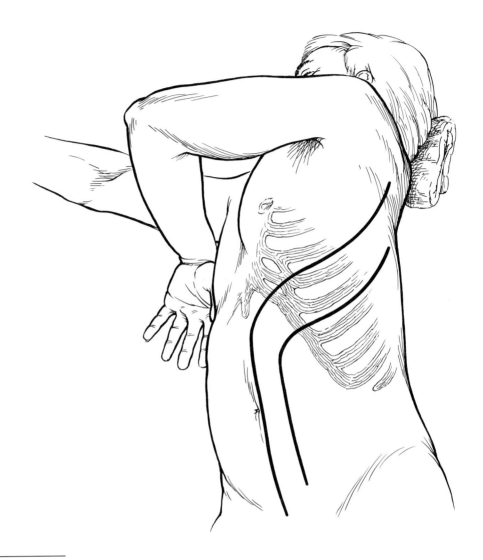

Figure 111

Options for thoracoabdominal aortic
exposure are shown. The upper sixth-rib
incision can be continued down the midline
of the abdomen; the eighth-rib incision can
be extended in a more lateral plane; or
modified combinations of these two
incisions may be performed, depending on
the extent of exposure required and the
desire to stay extraperitoneal.

Vascular Exposures

the suprarenal aorta but extending up into the lower thoracic aorta. It can also be used for antegrade aortomesenteric bypasses.

The eighth or ninth interspace incision crosses the costal margin but does not enter into the abdomen proper; that is, into the peritoneal sac (Fig. 112A). Instead, the left hemidiaphragm is divided and inch or so from its lateral insertion for at least three quarters of its circumference, extending from posteriorly at the left crus most of the way around to the midline anteriorly (Fig. 112B). By retracting downward and medially on the now freed up diaphragm, the retroperitoneum is entered posterolaterally, and then, with blunt dissection, mobilization and exposure proceed much as previously described for upper left retroperitoneal approaches, with the kidney and adrenal gland moved forward and the viscera enclosed within the peritoneal sac also mobilized anteriorly and medially. As seen in Figure 113, one eventually looks down on the distal thoracic and upper abdominal aorta from above, approaching the aorta on its posterolateral aspect. This exposure is excellent for transaortic endarterectomy for occlusive disease involving the suprarenal aorta and multiple orifices of the mesenteric and renal arteries, as well as suprarenal aneurysms. Professor Pokrovsky of the Vishnevsky Institute in Moscow has used it successfully for many years to deal with Takayasu's aortoarteritis involving this segment of the aorta. Closure requires reapproximation of the diaphragm (beginning with a few well-placed orienting sutures), followed by closing of the chest after insertion of a large, dependent chest tube.

Exposure of the Descending Thoracic Aorta. For diseases localized to the descending thoracic aorta (e.g., a localized aneurysm or an acquired coarctation secondary to Takayasu's aortoarteritis), one can employ a routine posterolateral thoracotomy through the sixth to eighth interspaces, the level being adjusted to center over the disease. For traumatic false aneurysms that involve the upper descending thoracic aorta just below the subclavian artery origin (typically of those caused by high-speed, decelerating injuries), one should move the incision up to at least the fifth rib or fourth interspace. The anatomy exposed by these thoracotomy incisions at different levels will not be separately shown here because the illustrations of thoracoabdominal exposures based on the same interspaces that follow provide much the same basic perspective.

Thoracoabdominal Aortic Exposures. The infrarenal aorta and its bifurcation is a site of predilection for both atherosclerotic occlusive and aneurysmal disease. As the disease progresses upward above the renal arteries, it can be reached through the direct transabdominal or left retroperitoneal approaches previously described, by mobilizing and retracting the viscera medially. But as the extent of the aortic disease—usually aneurysmal involvement—extends even higher, not only is thoracotomy inevitable but, with disease also involving the aorta below the renal arteries, some abdominal exposure is required and this may need to be extended downward as well. In extended thoracoabdominal exposures, after opening the sixth interspace or removing the sixth rib subperiosteally (the author's preference to obtain wider exposure without rib fracture), the abdomen is opened longitudinally, either by splitting the left rectus muscle or staying pararectus, as in the Risberg incision, or moving farther to the right and opening along the midline (see Fig. 111).

At the junction between the thoracotomy and celiotomy portions of the incision, it is wise to leave a few well-placed orienting sutures at equivalent locations along adjacent edges of the major layers that merge here; otherwise it

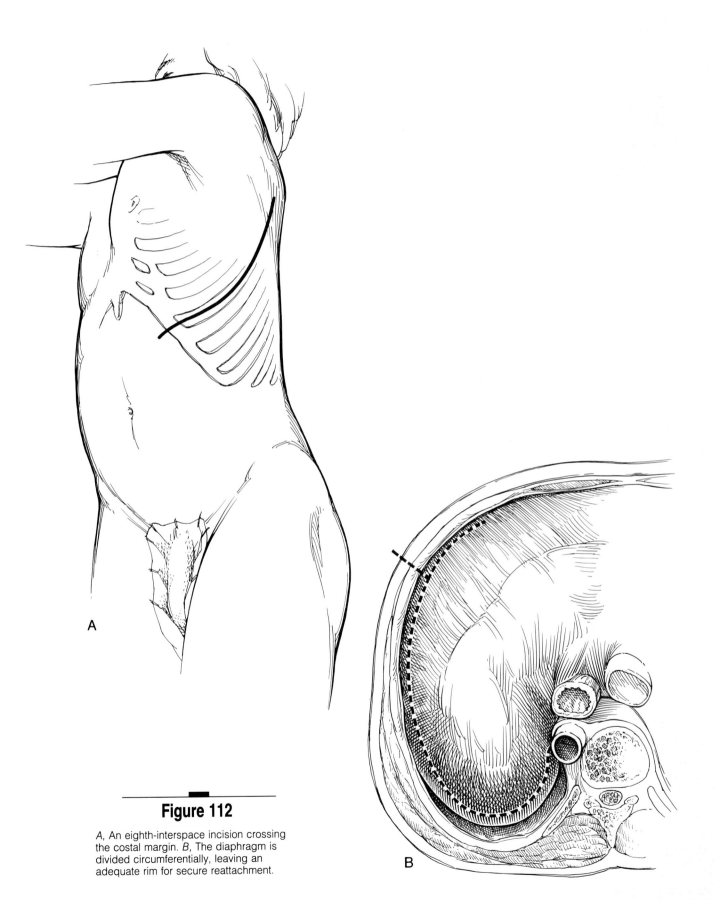

Figure 112

A, An eighth-interspace incision crossing the costal margin. B, The diaphragm is divided circumferentially, leaving an adequate rim for secure reattachment.

A

B

Vascular Exposures

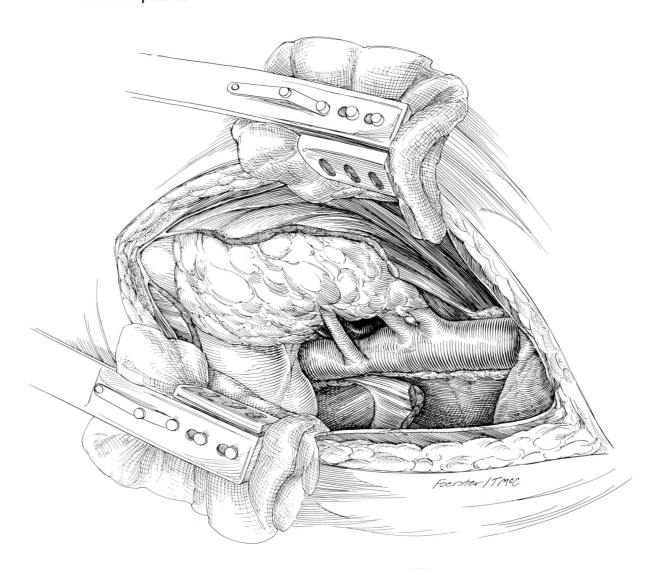

Figure 113

The final exposure obtained,
transthoracically and retroperitoneally, of the
distal thoracic and upper abdominal aorta.

is surprisingly easy to approximate these structures unevenly at the time of closure. In the open approach (sixth rib thoracotomy plus midline abdominal incision) the diaphragm can be opened radially between major vessels and nerves down to the crus overlying the aorta (Fig. 114*A* and *B*), and the viscera are rotated medially and held there with large self-retaining retractors.

This "medial viscera rotation" is easier than when performed through a midline abdominal incision alone. One is approaching the upper abdominal viscera posterolaterally rather than anteriorly. The length and breadth of the incision facilitate shifting the viscera to the right. This can provide exposure from the descending thoracic aorta down to the aortic bifurcation (Fig. 114*C*). For higher exposure, up to the subclavian artery, the lung can be retracted away from the overlying aorta, especially if one uses a Carlens endotracheal catheter to allow the left lung to be deflated. It may or may not be necessary to divide the inferior pulmonary ligament. By staying posteriorly, the vagus nerves can easily be avoided. Larger thoracic aneurysms may have induced pulmonary adhesions but these are usually easily separated. With division of the left crus of the diaphragm, this posterolateral exposure of the entire aorta is readily extended down into the abdomen.

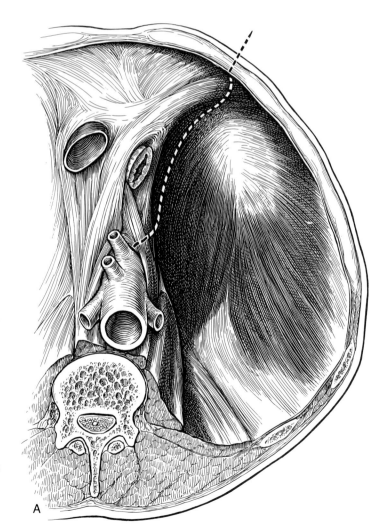

Figure 114

A, For wide transabdominal exposure, the diaphragm is divided radially. *B*, Cutting the diaphragm for open thoracoabdominal exposure. *C*, Exposure of the aorta from its bifurcation up to the mid-descending thoracic aorta.

A

Vascular Exposures

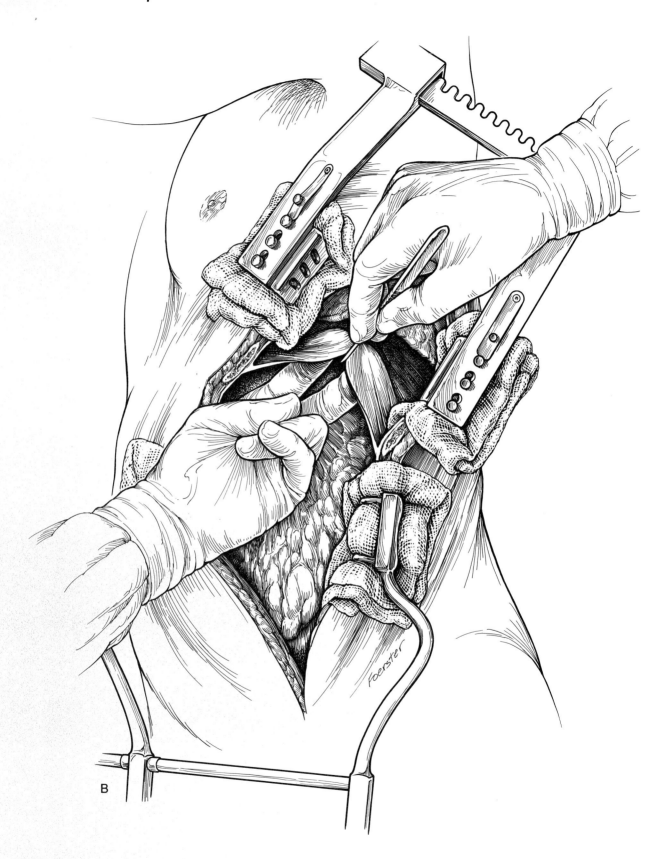

Foerster

B

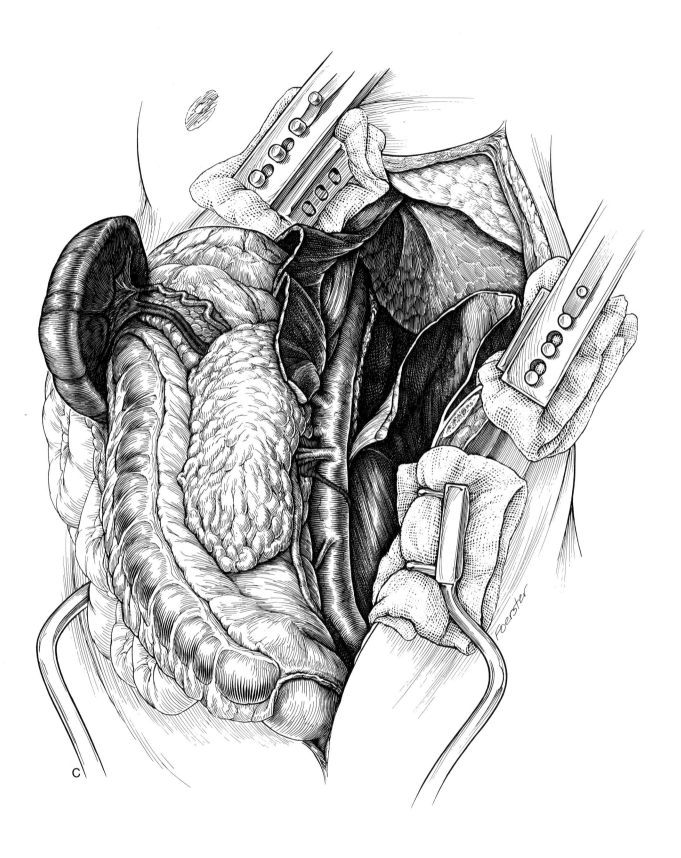

Vascular Exposures

Often, when dealing with aneurysmal disease beginning in the descending thoracic aorta, the disease extends to involve the suprarenal abdominal aorta but not beyond. In such a case, the chest is widely opened but only the upper abdomen is exposed (Fig. 115). If desired, one can even remain extraperitoneal by cutting the diaphragm circumferentially and proceeding much as described in Figures 112 and 113. In other instances, the aorta is involved all the way to the aortic bifurcation. Here the abdomen must be widely opened onto the lower abdomen with complete medial viscera rotation, allowing posterolateral exposure of the aorta all the way down to its bifurcation. In gaining this additional exposure, there is a structure that must be handled with caution—the left descending lumbar vein. This is a tributary of the left renal vein, which is thin walled and easily injured. As the kidney is retracted forward, it may be put under tension, which may attenuate or empty it, so that it may not seem impressively large or even may not be seen. It should be specifically sought, identified, and carefully divided between ligatures to allow continued forward retraction of the kidney and ongoing exposure of the full length of the aorta along its posterolateral aspect. A few other vessels in this area may bleed when transected but, if one is working in the true retroperitoneal plane, these will be few and far between.

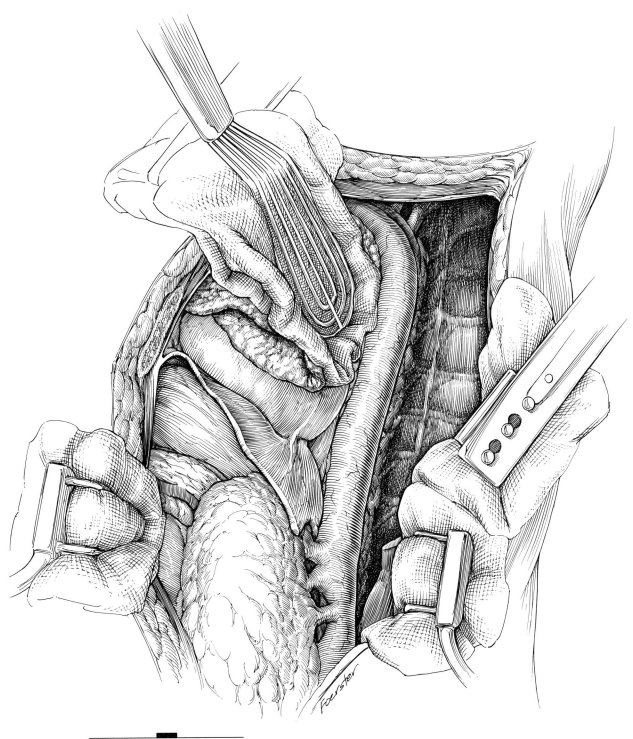

Figure 115

Exposure of the aorta from the left
subclavian artery to below the renal arteries.

Vascular Exposures

The ureter and gonadal vessels stay up with the peritoneal sac, as it is retracted upward and to the right. The left renal artery is readily seen just above the divided descending lumbar vein, for it will tend to angle outward before turning upward toward the kidney, especially if there is plaque near its origin and proximal segment. The superior mesenteric and celiac arteries, on the other hand, point directly anteriorly and are often not seen without deliberate dissection in that area. However, in most cases of aneurysmal disease it is not necessary that they be dissected, for they can be dealt with from inside the aorta. The inferior mesenteric artery, if patent, may be encountered exiting from the aorta in the lateral plane about one-third to one-half the way between the origin of the left common iliac artery and the left renal artery. The dissection plane stays behind the inferior mesenteric artery unless it is occluded, in which case it can be divided to aid in mobilization. Continuing distally, the posterolateral surface of the lower abdominal aorta runs almost imperceptively into the left common iliac artery. This artery is best encircled near its origin above the level where it is approached by the left iliac vein. Alternatively, one can move distally to the iliac bifurcation and, after mobilizing the ureter medially away from this area, the common iliac bifurcation can be isolated and controlled. The right iliac artery is more difficult to expose and control, so much so that, if the graft will terminate above the bifurcation, it is often simpler to control it from within after opening the aorta, with a 16F Foley catheter using a 30-cc balloon.

If *distal* control of the *right* iliac bifurcation is required, the left colon and sigmoid must be allowed to drop back to the left and the peritoneum overlying the iliac vessels incised and dissected just as previously described in Figure 90*A* and *B*. The final exposure of the thoracoabdominal aorta from the left subclavian to the left iliac arteries is seen in Figure 116.

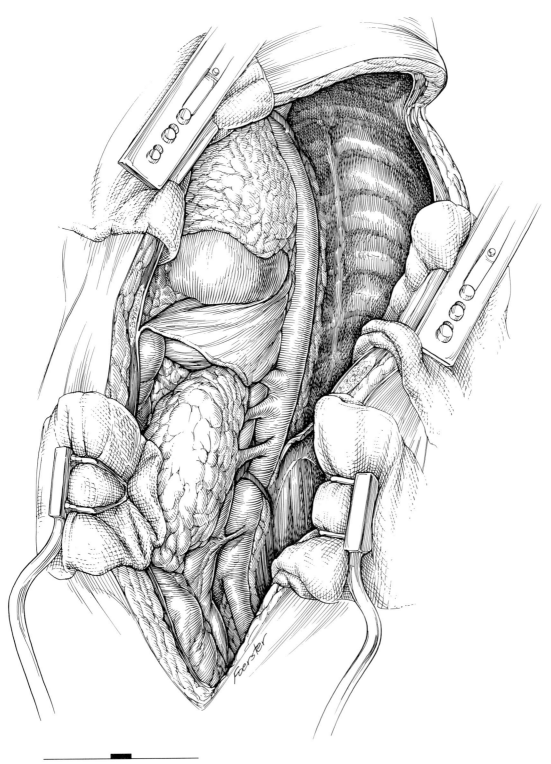

Figure 116

Exposure of the aorta from the left
subclavian artery to beyond its bifurcation.

EXPOSURE OF THE AORTIC ARCH AND BRACHIOCEPHALIC VESSELS (INCLUDING THE CAROTID ARTERIES)

The proximal left subclavian artery cannot readily be reached by a median sternotomy approach, as might be apparent from the upper descending thoracic aortic exposures featured at the end of the previous section. The left subclavian artery and its aortic origin can best be approached through a posterolateral thoracotomy, usually through the bed of a resected fourth rib or the fourth interspace. However, proximal to this point, the aortic arch and its other major branches can be more readily exposed by a median sternotomy with or without extensions up along the sternocleidomastoid muscles for carotid exposure or supraclavicular extensions for exposure of the subclavian vessels. These options are shown in Figure 117*A*.

Exposure of the Proximal and Middle Thirds of the Aortic Arch and the Innominate and Proximal Left Common Carotid Arteries. The patient should be supine with both arms appropriately cannulated for vascular access and then protected and positioned down by the sides. A transverse roll may be placed across the shoulders and the upper torso elevated about 10° to 15°, enough so that the sternum is at or slightly above the horizontal plane. The neck is slightly extended and the occiput rests on a "donut," with the head turned to one side if extension into the neck is anticipated. Unless extension into the neck is planned, however, the upper end of the median sternotomy incision can be crossed at the top, or "T-ed," to give equal upper exposure without an unsightly vertical lower cervical scar.

After the anterior surface of the sternum is exposed, the superior aspect is cleared off by blunt dissection as close to it as possible and then a sternotomy saw is inserted into this deepened plane. The sternotomy is performed after first cauterizing the anterior surface of the periosteum all the way down to the end of the sternum, the incision being carried off to one side of the xiphoid process (Fig. 117*B*). For limited upper exposures, or to begin a "book end" or "trap door" opening into one hemithorax, one can do a partial sternotomy, then open laterally into an interspace—usually the third. However, in most cases, it is better to complete the entire sternotomy. It is faster, is no more uncomfortable, and offers a much wider exposure and more secure closure.

Figure 117*C* shows the vascular exposure that can be obtained through this incision with little further dissection beyond the point of sternal retraction other than separating or excising the two lobes of the thymus overlying the left brachiocephalic vein. The triple arterial supply of each lobe of the thymus enters laterally and via both poles, so that the two lobes can be separated in the midline without concern for arterial supply. However, one or two small veins often drain from these lobes into the innominate (left brachiocephalic) vein. These should be looked for and divided; otherwise, they may tear and cause considerable bleeding. A tongue of pericardial sac reaches well up onto the anterior surface of the ascending aorta, and this must be dissected away to allow grafts to originate from this point. The left brachiocephalic vein lies in front of the origin of the innominate artery, but with a Silastic loop around it for traction it rarely needs to be divided to work on the latter vessel. One can work on either side of this vein and, if an aortoinnominate bypass is performed, it can pass underneath it.

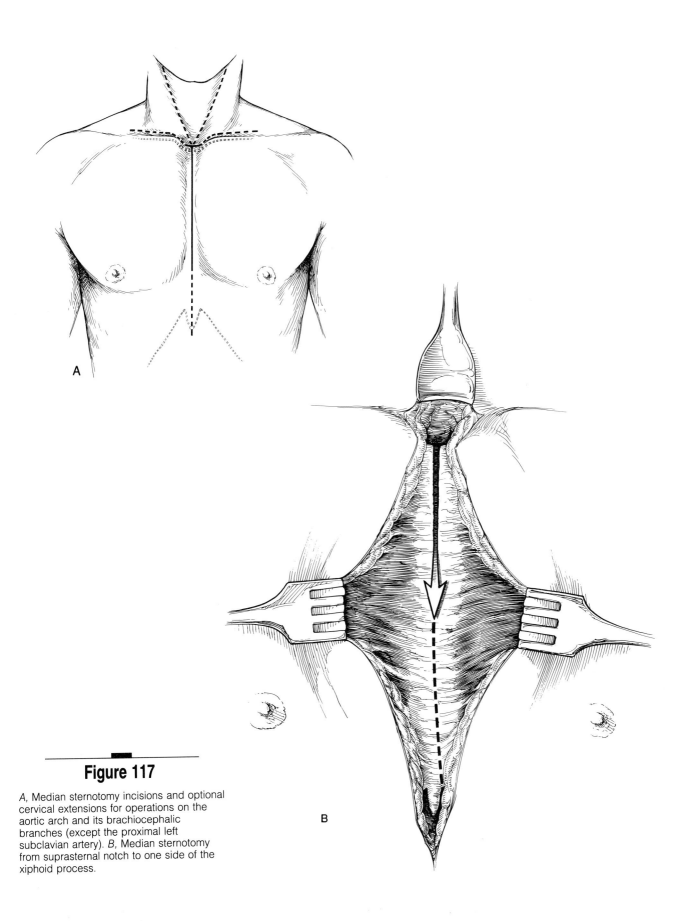

Figure 117

A, Median sternotomy incisions and optional cervical extensions for operations on the aortic arch and its brachiocephalic branches (except the proximal left subclavian artery). *B,* Median sternotomy from suprasternal notch to one side of the xiphoid process.

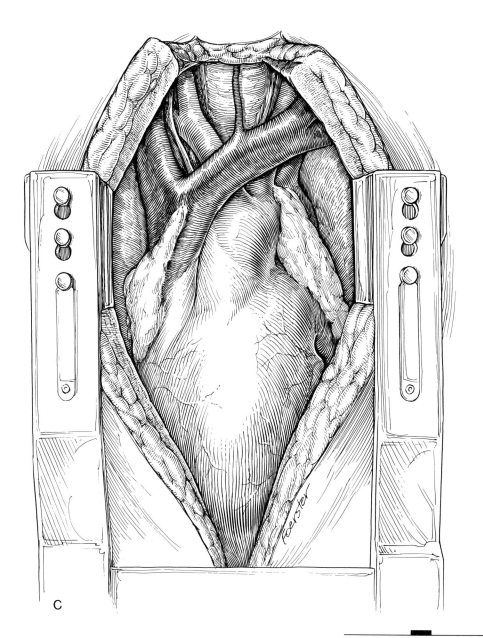

C

Figure 117 *Continued*

C, Final exposure through a median
sternotomy incision, with the thymus
removed for better visualization.

The proximal left common carotid artery is somewhat deeper but can be reached by this approach. However, clamp placement here can be made difficult by arteriosclerotic plaque spanning the roof of the aortic arch and extending up into the orifices of these vessels. The same can be said if a "bovine" aortic arch exists in which the innominate and left carotid arteries share a common origin, rendering them difficult to separate for clamping purposes. Fortunately, separate operations on the proximal (intrathoracic) portion of the left common carotid artery are rare. Occlusive disease there is usually dealt with by cervical bypass. The most common reason for vascular surgery using the aforementioned approach is to deal with disease at the origin of the innominate artery, which is usually managed by aorta-to-innominate bypass rather than by endarterectomy.

Extension of the sternotomy incision up along the anterior border of the sternocleidomastoid exposes the innominate bifurcation and the proximal inch or two of the right subclavian and carotid arteries. For this exposure the internal jugular vein is retracted laterally, and here one must be careful to protect the right vagus nerve crossing over the anterior surface of the subclavian as well as the recurrent laryngeal nerve, which leaves the vagus here and curls backward under the subclavian artery to ascend into the neck again. The proximal *left* common carotid artery lies deeper than the innominate artery and is often obscured by the left brachiocephalic vein. Lateral retraction of the vein is difficult because it is held in place by its internal jugular tributary. It is not often one needs to expose the *origin* of the left common carotid artery. Bypass grafts from the aorta, or from other arch vessels to the left common carotid artery, would usually be placed higher up on this vessel where, after extending the thoracotomy incision up along the anterior border of the sternocleidomastoid muscle, it can be readily found just medial to the internal jugular vein.

Carotid Artery Exposure

Exposure of the Common Carotid Artery Bifurcation and the Upper Internal Carotid Artery. The common incision for carotid endarterectomy is described. The patient lies supine with the head turned to the opposite side. The opposite upper extremity should be used for both an intravenous access and a monitoring arterial cannula. This, along with bringing the connecting tubing from the endotracheal tube down to the same side, allows the anesthesiologist to be stationed there, next to the patient's wrist, rather than at the head of the table. The surgeon and first assistant can stand opposite each other, with the second assistant at the head of the table. Not only does this arrangement provide room for the additional assistant but also it avoids having this person come between the operating team and the scrub nurse and instrument stand. If the operating table is turned 90°, this positioning can occur without needing to move the anesthesiologists and their equipment and monitoring consoles. The table should be tilted away from the surgeon so that the operative field (side of the neck) is brought into a more horizontal plane.

Vascular Exposures

Figure 118*A* shows the location of the incision, along the anterior border of the sternocleidomastoid muscle, roughly the upper two thirds of the distance from its insertion to its origin. The level of the carotid artery bifurcation may vary, as may the distance arteriosclerotic plaque extends up into the internal carotid artery. Reference to a lateral arteriographic view of the carotid bifurcation, noting its position relative to the angle of the mandible or the C-2 vertebra, provides a valuable perspective. Disease higher than this may well require special additional steps in exposure, to be discussed later.

For the usual anatomy, the incision need not reach any higher than the tip of the ear lobe. Once the skin, subcutaneous tissue, and platysma have been incised, the incision is deepened directly in front of the sternocleidomastoid muscle for the length of the incision. This exposes the internal jugular vein, allowing one to proceed in front of that vein to reach the carotid artery. As seen on the cross-sectional view (Fig. 118*B*), this leads into the carotid artery in a plane *behind* (posterior to) the vascular lymph node–bearing tissues that lie over the carotid bifurcation. Annoying bleeding from these structures may be encountered if one dissects directly inward toward the palpable carotid pulse. Furthermore, if higher exposure is needed, it is best to obtain this by dissecting up along the cleft between the internal jugular vein and the internal carotid artery. Therefore, exposing the internal jugular as part of the dissection has additional advantages.

For full exposure, the anterior borders of the sternocleidomastoid muscle and then the internal jugular vein are exposed from the omohyoid muscle below to the lower edge of the parotid gland above. This will expose the common facial vein, as it drains into the anterior aspect of the internal jugular vein (Fig. 118*C*). It frequently lies directly over the carotid bifurcation and should be divided between heavy ligatures. The ansa hypoglossi nerve is usually encountered at this point just under the divided common facial vein. Although it can be divided without noticeable penalty, it may be preserved by dissecting *posterior* to it to reach the carotid artery. This will also allow it to serve as a guide to the position of the hypoglossal nerve, as the dissection proceeds upward. By mobilizing both of these nerves forward, even higher exposure can be obtained, if needed (see later).

The sheath over the common carotid artery low in the field is opened. The common carotid artery is encircled with an umbilical tape to which a Rummel tourniquet can be affixed, in case a temporary indwelling shunt is needed. Then, proceeding upward from there, the carotid bifurcation is approached and, as soon as feasible, the carotid sinus nerve, deep in the crotch between the internal and external carotid arteries, is anesthetized by injecting it with Xylocaine (lidocaine) (Fig. 118*D*). If not, mobilization of the carotid bifurcation will cause afferent impulses to be relayed up the sinus nerve to the hypoglossal nerve, with a reflex arc relayed down the vagus nerve to produce severe bradycardia and hypotension. After mobilizing the common carotid artery and defunctionalizing the sinus nerve, attention should be turned to the external carotid artery. At its base the first branch, the superior thyroid artery, is usually separately encircled with a heavy silk Potts loop for control. The external carotid artery above it is then mobilized and encircled with an umbilical tape and a Rummel tourniquet. The internal carotid artery is approached well above the bifurcation in a palpably soft segment. Once the sheath around it is opened, dissection proceeds quite easily and the artery is encircled, staying close to its adventitial surface. This dissection attempts to disturb the bifurcation and proximal internal artery as little as possible until control has been obtained, to avoid inducing embolism from atheromatous plaques there. The final exposure is seen in Figure 118*E*.

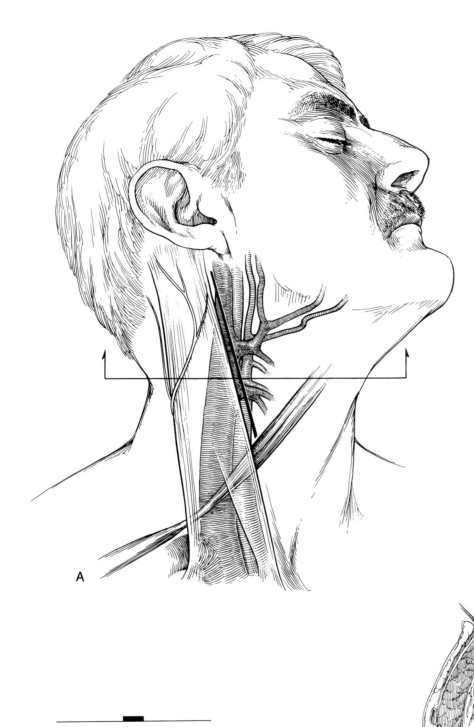

A

B

Figure 118

A, Common incision for carotid endarterectomy, along the upper two thirds of the anterior border of the sternocleidomastoid muscle. *B,* Cross section showing the preferred route into the carotid bifurcation, immediately in front of the sternocleidomastoid muscle and internal jugular vein, to avoid most of the overlying cluster of lymph nodes.

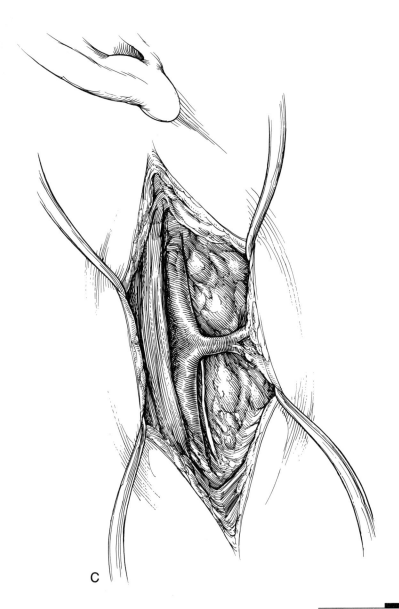

C

Figure 118 *Continued*

C, With the sternocleidomastoid muscle and internal jugular vein exposed from the tip of the parotid gland above to the omohyoid muscle below, only the common facial vein bars the way into the carotid bifurcation. *D,* As soon as the bifurcation is sufficiently exposed, the sinus nerve, deep in the crotch of the bifurcation, is injected with a local anesthetic. *E,* Rumel tourniquets are placed around each of the three carotid arteries to facilitate shunt placement. The usual positions of the vagus nerve, the hypoglossal nerve, and the ansa hypoglossi are shown.

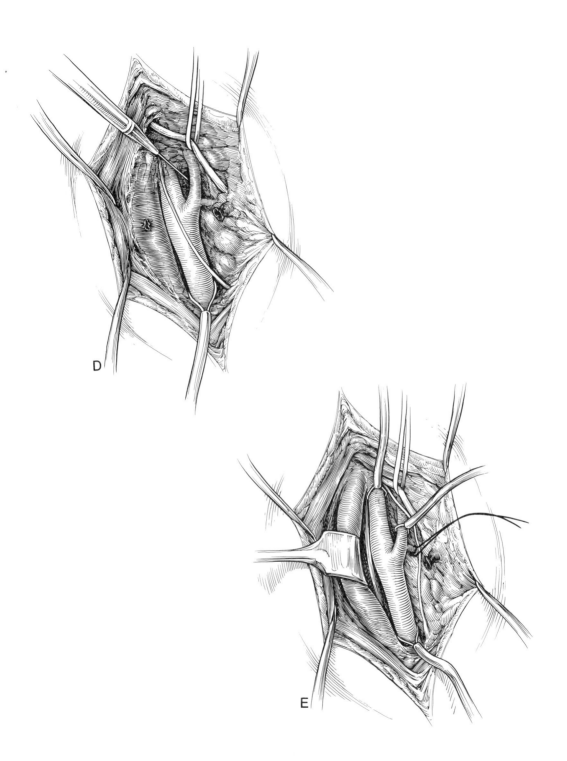

Vascular Exposures

Obtaining Higher Exposure of the Internal Carotid Artery. This can be obtained in increments through a number of stepwise maneuvers. First, one procceds upward in the space between the internal jugular vein and internal carotid artery. If not already seen, the hypoglossal nerve will be encountered here with the ansa hypoglossi leading up to it. They come close together high in the neck and, importantly, at this point are usually tethered down by vessels to the sternocleidomastoid muscle, which loop around them. These vessels have to be divided to free these nerves and mobilize them forward to allow dissection to continue upward. At this point, if still further upward exposure is needed, the posterior belly of the digastric muscle can be divided. Beyond this, further exposure is difficult without retracting the mandible forward. This is done with difficulty because the retractor usually takes up as much space as it gains. However, if one anticipates this need, one can have the temporomandibular joints subluxated (not dislocated) forward. This can be performed at the beginning of the operation after anesthetizing the patient, deliberately using nasotracheal intubation. This forward position can be sustained by heavy wires placed around the mandible and through the maxilla, coming out through the nares. These are pulled together by twisting on a third, traction suture (Fig. 119*A*). Alternatively, if time allows preoperatively, patients with teeth can be sent to a dentist or oral surgeon, where a simple mold can be made with the teeth held voluntarily in this prognathic position, avoiding the need for wiring at the time of operation. Nasotracheal intubation will be required, but at least the jaws can be simply bound in position over this mold without the need for wires.

Cutting the stylohyoid tendon and applying a rongeur to the stylohyoid process adds some additional exposure but, at this point, the risk of serious nerve injury becomes a significant deterrent. This can be appreciated from studying Figure 119*A*. Although injuries to the lower branch of the facial, hypoglossal, spinal accessory, and vagus nerves and, directly or indirectly, the superior and recurrent laryngeal nerves have all been reported in most large, carefully documented series, the most disastrous of all the cranial nerve injuries associated with carotid artery surgery is to the glossopharyngeal nerve, for it often results in permanent tracheostomy. The glossopharyngeal nerve lies high up along the inner aspect of the internal carotid artery. Although it is not usually directly visualized, it is deliberately shown in the final illustration of high carotid exposure (Fig. 119*B*).

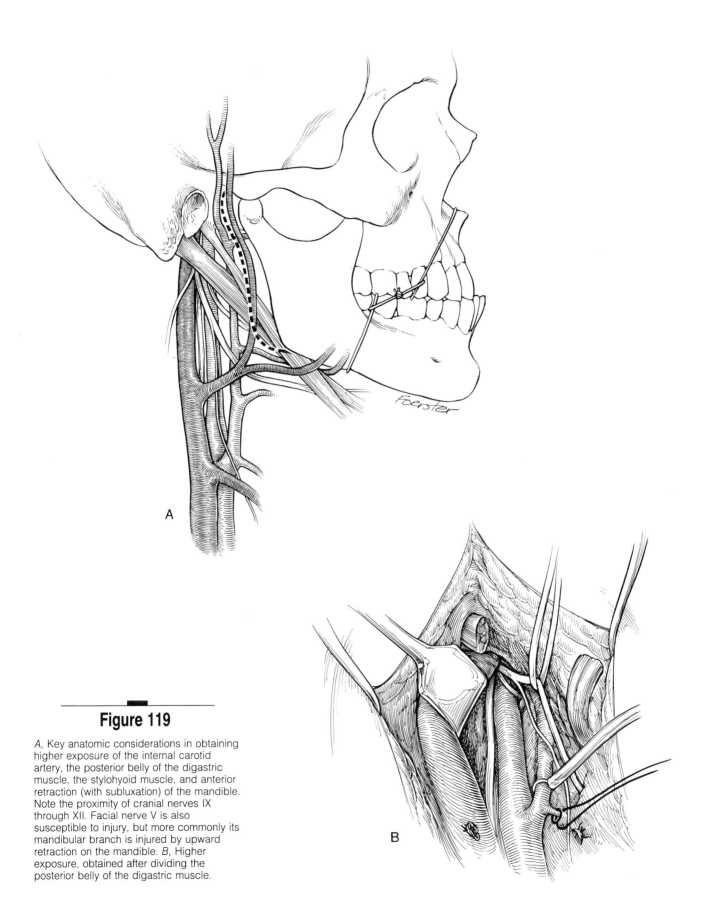

Figure 119

A, Key anatomic considerations in obtaining higher exposure of the internal carotid artery, the posterior belly of the digastric muscle, the stylohyoid muscle, and anterior retraction (with subluxation) of the mandible. Note the proximity of cranial nerves IX through XII. Facial nerve V is also susceptible to injury, but more commonly its mandibular branch is injured by upward retraction on the mandible. *B,* Higher exposure, obtained after dividing the posterior belly of the digastric muscle.

Vascular Exposures

Supraclavicular Exposures

The subclavian artery and its branches (particularly the proximal vertebral artery), the common carotid artery, and the accompanying major veins, as well as the cervicothoracic sympathetic chain, can all be exposed using minor variations of the same basic supraclavicular incision. This exposure allows such procedures as carotid subclavian bypass or transposition, vertebral artery transposition, dorsal sympathectomy, and—using a more limited incision—exposure of the internal jugular vein for angioaccess and caval filter placement to be performed.

On the left side, the subclavian vessels are relatively more deeply placed and one must also contend with the thoracic duct. Right-sided supraclavicular exposure is illustrated because of the additional exposure of the upper innominate artery it allows. The patient lies supine with the head turned to the opposite side. The arm is down at the side with the shoulder depressed as much as possible. The supraclavicular incision is made about 1 FB above the upper edge of the clavicle. Its medial and lateral extensions will be determined by the particular vascular structures to be exposed. A short incision centered over the two heads of the sternocleidomastoid muscles will expose the internal jugular vein or common carotid artery. An incision across the lateral head of the sternocleidomastoid muscle, extending an equal distance laterally, can expose both the subclavian artery and its branches as well as the carotid artery and the sympathetic chain. This is the most common incision used.

On the right side, a further medial extension across the medial head of the sternocleidomastoid and into the suprasternal notch, after division of both heads of that muscle and the underlying strap muscles, will allow the distal innominate artery to be included in the field, without the need for splitting the sternum. Finally, one can curve the medial aspect of this supraclavicular incision up along the anterior border of the sternocleidomastoid muscle to include higher segments of the carotid and jugular vessels. For an internal jugular "turn down" to anastomose to the axillary vein, this extension must often be carried all the way up to the mastoid process. These variations, including a cross-clavicle incision for removing that bone and gaining both supraclavicular and infraclavicular exposure, are shown in Figure 120.

For the usual supraclavicular exposure, after dividing the platysma and lateral head of the sternocleidomastoid muscle, the omohyoid is identified, elevated, and divided (Fig. 121*A*). The prescalene fat pad then lies exposed. It is dissected upward by freeing it along its medial and inferior surfaces so that it can be ultimately retracted upward and laterally out of the way. This exposes the underlying anterior scalene muscle with the phrenic nerve usually lying along its medial aspect, encroaching on its anterior surface increasingly as one proceeds distally. Although accessory branches of the phrenic nerve are not uncommon, it should be assumed that this nerve is the only innervation of the hemidiaphragm, particularly if it is found in this, its most common position. Therefore, it should be handled with extreme caution. Some warn against any retraction on it, but gentle retraction by a thin Silastic loop is useful while the anterior scalene muscle is being divided. This should be done as close to its insertion as possible and may be done in piecemeal fashion, using Metzenbaum scissors. In most cases, if the nerve is retracted out of the way and the fibers are lifted up with a blunt right-angle clamp, cautery division, using the lowest current, is safe (Fig. 121*B*).

After the anterior scalene muscle has been divided, the pulse of the subclavian artery will usually be felt directly below in the bottom of the wound but it is covered by a fascial layer. Once this has been opened, the subclavian artery can be dissected free and encircled at its most superior point or apex. The lower cords of the brachial plexus lie a little higher in the neck than the artery, laterally and in a slightly deeper plane at this point. With traction on the apex of the subclavian artery, it can then be progressively mobilized, proceeding medially (Fig. 121C). The thyrocervical trunk is encountered first; then, moving medially, the internal mammary artery will be found anteriorly, and pointing cardiad and just medial to this, but posterior and aiming cephalad, is the vertebral artery. These branches may be encircled, and proximal control of the subclavian artery is usually obtained just proximal to their origins (Fig. 121D).

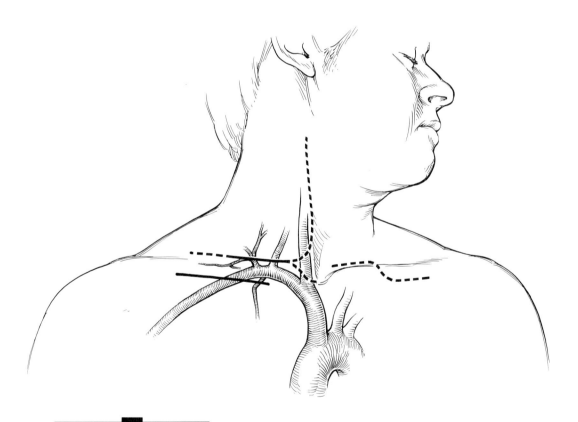

Figure 120

A number of incisions are shown for exposing the subclavian and axillary vessels, along with an extension upward to include the carotid artery or internal jugular vein and a cross clavicular incision used when removing the clavicle.

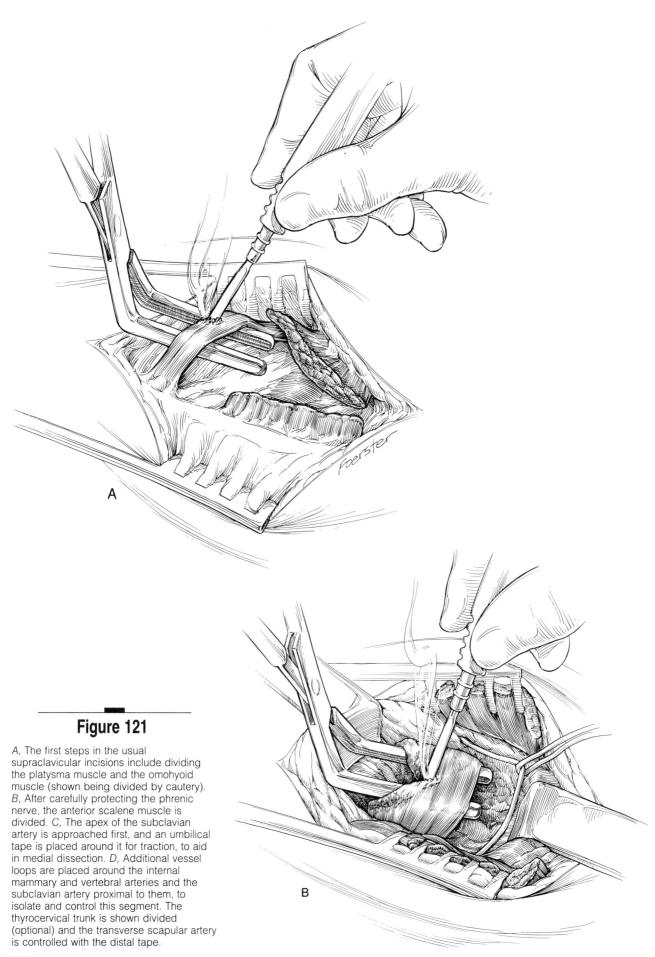

A

B

Figure 121

A, The first steps in the usual
supraclavicular incisions include dividing
the platysma muscle and the omohyoid
muscle (shown being divided by cautery).
B, After carefully protecting the phrenic
nerve, the anterior scalene muscle is
divided. *C,* The apex of the subclavian
artery is approached first, and an umbilical
tape is placed around it for traction, to aid
in medial dissection. *D,* Additional vessel
loops are placed around the internal
mammary and vertebral arteries and the
subclavian artery proximal to them, to
isolate and control this segment. The
thyrocervical trunk is shown divided
(optional) and the transverse scapular artery
is controlled with the distal tape.

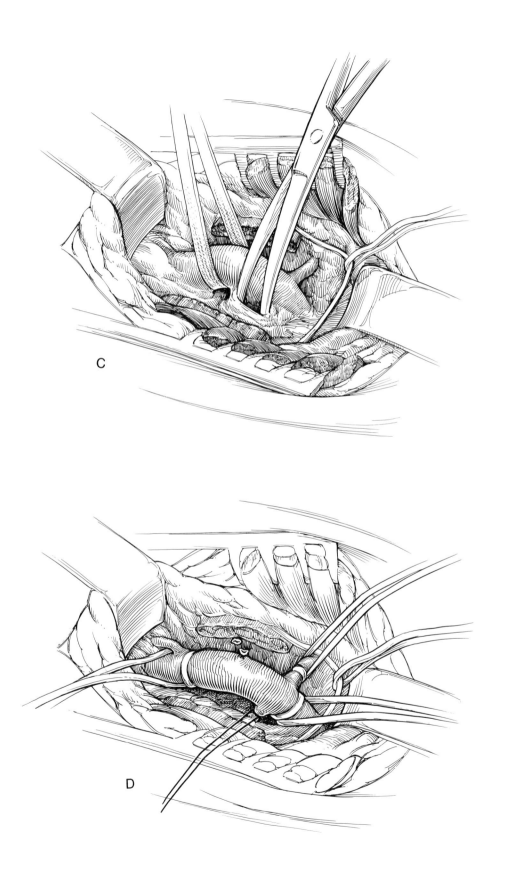

C

D

Vascular Exposures

Feeling with the fingertip just below and medial to the vertebral artery, on the rim of the thoracic inlet and right on the neck of the first rib, one will detect the unmistakable firm snapping sensation of stroking across the stellate ganglion. Higher in the middle of the field and medially, exposed when the lateral head of the sternocleidomastoid muscle is divided, is the internal jugular vein. The carotid artery lies just medial and deep to this vein, with the vagus nerve coursing between them (Fig. 122). Even on the right side, a major lymphatic tributary enters near the confluence of the internal jugular and subclavian veins. On the left side, this is the thoracic duct and, if injured, it should be deliberately ligated rather than risk a lymph fistula.

On the right side, to expose the remainder of the proximal portions of the common carotid and subclavian arteries, and to reach to the distal innominate artery, the internal jugular vein bars the way (Fig. 123A). It may be retracted in one direction or the other and one can work around it for limited procedures, but, if the entire subclavian artery is to be exposed all the way down to the upper innominate artery, it may simply be divided. After this, the strap muscles must also be divided to reach the proximal innominate artery. Mobilization of the proximal subclavian artery is made more difficult by the overlying vagus nerve and the recurrent laryngeal nerve that loops around it from anterior to posterior (Fig. 123B).

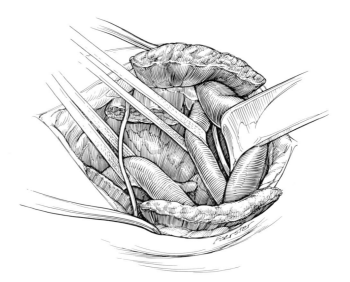

Figure 122

If carotid exposure and control are also required through this incision, the artery can be found with the vagus nerve just below the jugular vein, as shown.

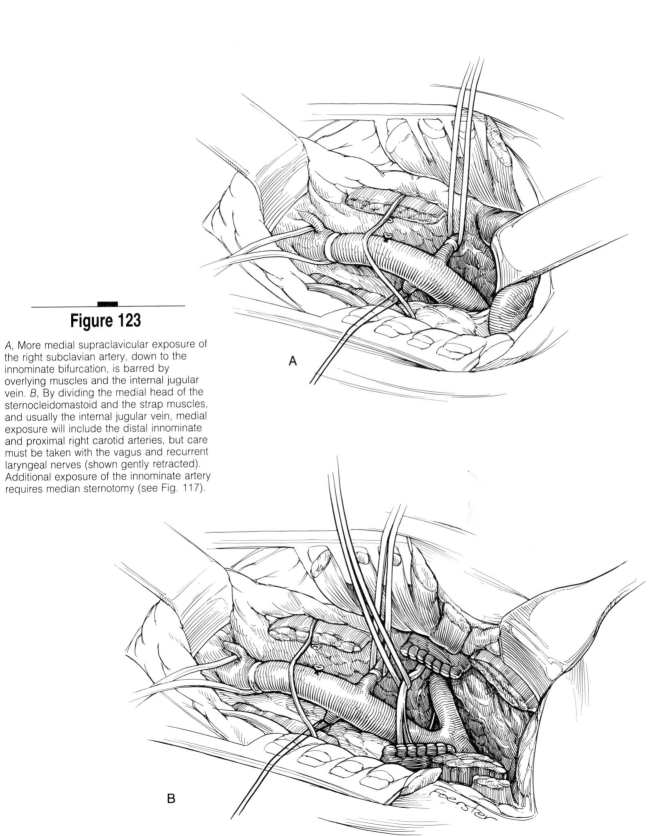

Figure 123

A, More medial supraclavicular exposure of the right subclavian artery, down to the innominate bifurcation, is barred by overlying muscles and the internal jugular vein. *B,* By dividing the medial head of the sternocleidomastoid and the strap muscles, and usually the internal jugular vein, medial exposure will include the distal innominate and proximal right carotid arteries, but care must be taken with the vagus and recurrent laryngeal nerves (shown gently retracted). Additional exposure of the innominate artery requires median sternotomy (see Fig. 117).

Vascular Exposures

Infraclavicular Exposures

Infraclavicular Exposure of the Axillary Vessels. Positioning of the arm and shoulder is important in exposing the axillary vessels. Although it might seem that having the arm out to the side at 90° is ideal (and it has certain advantages if other incisions will be made distally on the arm for bypass or for multiple-site thromboembolectomies), that position has the disadvantage, when approaching the axillary vessels, of pulling them downward, deeper into the axilla, and away from the skin surface. Therefore, as suggested by Kaj Johansen, if only the axillary artery requires exposure, as in an axillobifemoral bypass, a better position for the arm is with the hand down to the side with the elbow slightly flexed, almost as if the hand were being placed in an imaginary pants pocket. The opposite arm is used for angioaccess for arterial monitoring and intravenous infusions. To allow the first assistant better opportunity to work, the patient's upper body should be elevated 10° to 15° and tilted toward the opposite side so that the skin of the overlying infraclavicular fossa is close to a horizontal plane.

The incision is usually made from a point just lateral to the sternal head of the clavicle, over to the top of the deltopectoral groove, beginning 1 FB below the clavicle and ending about 2 FB below the clavicle (Fig. 124A). One may try to enter between the sternal and clavicular heads of the pectoralis major if the line of separation is apparent, but it is appropriate to enter at any convenient point by splitting the fibers of this muscle.

As seen in Figure 124B, the pathway into the vessels then passes through the deltopectoral or (more correctly) clavipectoral fascia. If the approach is high enough, the cephalic vein may be followed down between the two heads of the pectoralis muscle to where it penetrates the fascia to join the axillary vein. A few small vessels cross the field there just under the fascia and are visible through it.

Figure 124C shows these relationships and the pectoralis minor muscle, which lies just under the fascia in the lateral aspect of the wound. The pectoralis minor muscle is actually partly enveloped by that fascia and will be seen as soon as the fascia is opened, its fibers slanting downward and inward. Arterial branches of the thoracoacromial trunk and their accompanying veins will be encountered. They may be divided as necessary to gain full entry through the fatty tissue overlying the axillary vessels. Following one of these arterial branches down will often lead one right to the thoracoacromial trunk and thus to the most appropriate segment of the axillary artery to be exposed.

In most instances, division of the pectoralis minor muscle greatly facilitates exposure and, in the case of axillofemoral bypass, allows the graft to be tunneled down the side of the thorax without impingement. This is best done as high as possible, where the muscle is narrower and more tendinous, cauterizing it over a finger slipped underneath it at this point (Fig. 124D). One should remember that the pectoralis minor muscle usually has a vessel running along its lateral edge.

In this dissection, one will often encounter one of the two nerves to the pectoralis major muscle and these should be preserved, if possible, particularly in younger patients. By gently dissecting away the overlying fat, the axillary vein is usually encountered first. The axillary artery lies superior and deep to the vein and, if patent, is readily palpated. If approached directly, using nearby branches of the thoracoacromial trunk to guide the downward dissection, the artery can be readily exposed and, using a right-angle clamp, encircled with an umbilical tape. This maneuver will allow the axillary artery to be drawn up into the wound away from the cords of the brachial plexus superiorly and the axillary vein inferiorly (Fig. 124E). One or two venous tributaries may need to be divided between ligatures to allow the artery to be drawn up into the wound. If the artery is to be used for an end-to-side bypass anastomosis, as is most commonly the case, the thoracoacromial trunk can be divided and the artery encircled by tapes and elevated into the wound for easier access. Final exposure is seen in Figure 124*F*.

If the axillary vein is the focus of attention, as in subclavian-axillary thrombectomy, it can be mobilized without disturbing the artery, from its major deep branch up to just above the point of entry of the cephalic vein, using this same basic exposure. To gain higher exposure, the subclavius muscle will need to be divided. Beyond this, the medial half of the clavicle must be resected to gain access to its confluence with the internal jugular vein.

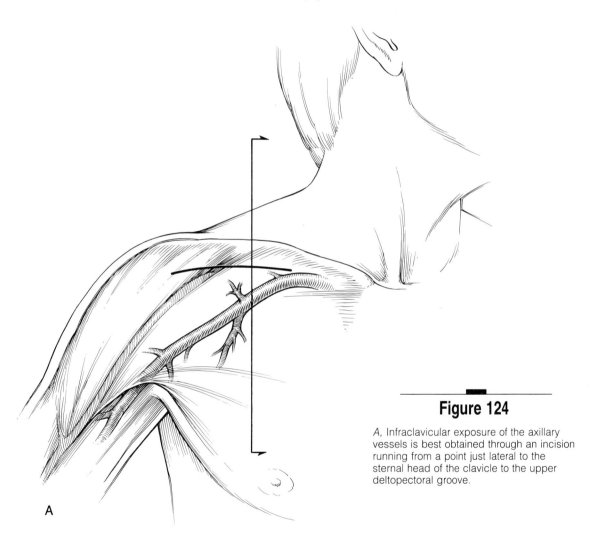

Figure 124

A, Infraclavicular exposure of the axillary vessels is best obtained through an incision running from a point just lateral to the sternal head of the clavicle to the upper deltopectoral groove.

A

Vascular Exposures

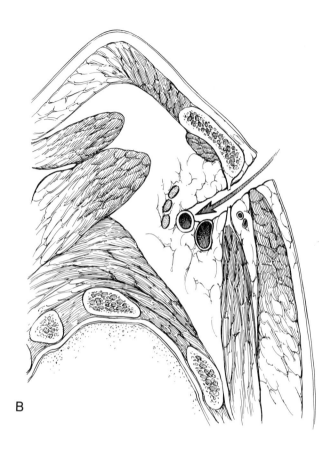

B

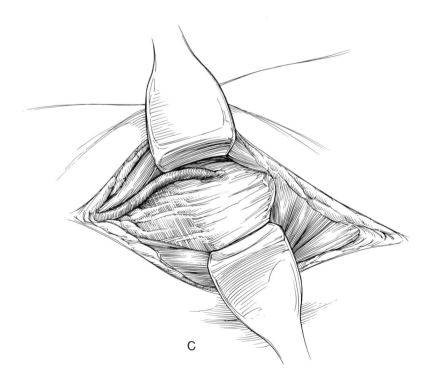

C

Figure 124 *Continued*

B, Cross-sectional view shows the route into the axillary vessels, past the pectoral muscles and clavipectoral fascia, with the relative positions of the axillary vein and cords of the brachial plexus. *C,* After the fibers of the pectoralis major muscle have been separated, the clavipectoral fascia is encountered, with the pectoralis minor muscle lying in the lateral half of the incision. The cephalic vein may be encountered, as it drops down between the two heads of the pectoralis major to join the axillary vein. *D,* After opening the clavipectoral fascia, branches of the thoracoacromial trunk will be encountered, leading to the axillary artery. The pectoralis minor muscle usually must be divided, as shown. *E,* The thoracoacromial trunk marks the best location for anastomosis and is usually divided. A traction tape placed early around the axillary artery aids dissection. *F,* Final exposure of the axillary artery.

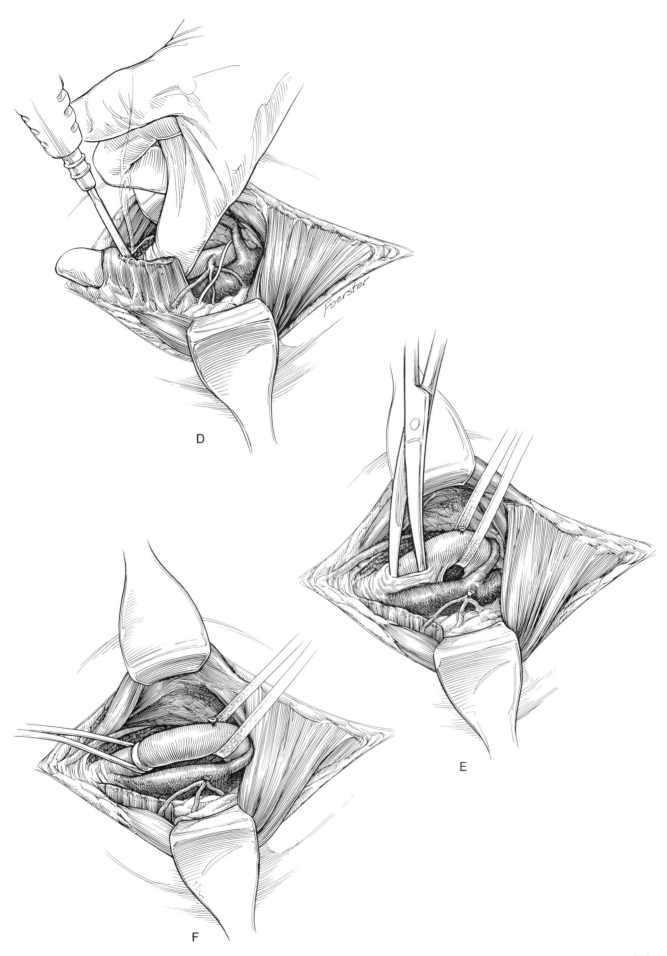

D

E

F

EXPOSURES OF THE UPPER EXTREMITY ARTERIES

The common exposures employed in the arm itself, shown in Figure 125, are extensile. In the upper arm they extend in a straight line over the brachial vessels from the axilla to just above the elbow. The upper end of the incision can be carried up onto the shoulder, along the deltopectoral groove and, if needed, continued to include the supraclavicular exposure of the proximal axillary vessels just described. This extension is sometimes valuable in dealing with vascular injuries but is rarely needed in elective reconstructions. In the latter circumstance, one can work around the insertion of the sternal head of the pectoralis major muscle or divide and reattach it, being cautious not to damage the musculocutaneous nerve, which is surprisingly vulnerable here.

Exposure of the brachial artery along its upper course is made by longitudinal incision, opening the sheath surrounding the neurovascular bundle and carefully dissecting the artery away from the accompanying basilic vein and venae comitantes and the adjacent nerves, especially the median nerve that lies just posteromedial to it. In primary elective operations, this is a simple task. In reoperations or explorations for trauma, including hematoma following transaxillary arteriography, the anatomy may be obscured by blood or scar, and no illustration could do it justice. One can only dissect carefully, in a longitudinal direction, being mindful of the proximity of the median and ulnar nerves.

The most common exposure of the brachial artery is performed distally at its bifurcation. This is a site of iatrogenic trauma, at the time of cardiac catheterization, and a preferred point of approach to retrieve distal emboli because balloon catheters can be guided into both radial and ulnar arteries from above at this point. It is also a common site for angioaccess shunts or fistulas, or both, but in these operations, shorter transverse incisions just above or below the antecubital crease are preferred. As shown in Figure 126*A,* the longitudinal incision includes a short transverse segment as it crosses the crease, much as employed with posterior exposure of the popliteal artery. As shown in Figure 126*B,* not only the overlying fascia but also the fibrous extensions of the biceps tendon must be divided, along with a major antecubital connection to the basilic vein. The brachial artery is best exposed first just above the elbow, while remembering the nearness of the median nerve just medial to it. Using traction on the brachial artery and following it down, the ulnar and radial branches are progressively exposed and looped. In controlling the latter, the branch of the radial nerve to the brachioradialis muscle must be protected. Final exposure is seen in Figure 126*C.*

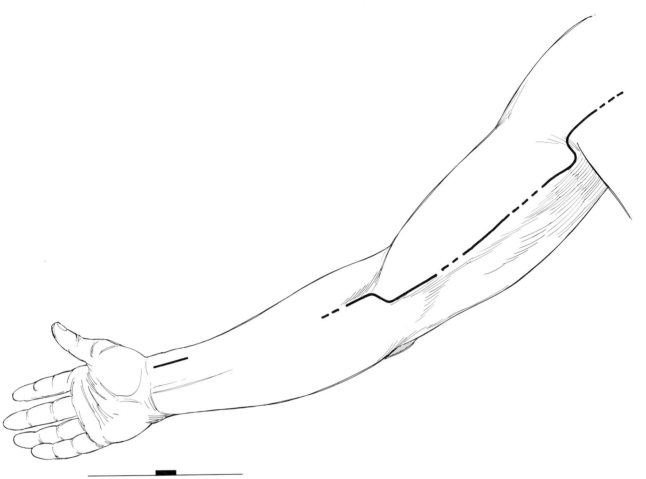

Figure 125

The right upper extremity, showing a
number of extensile exposures placed along
the arterial tree.

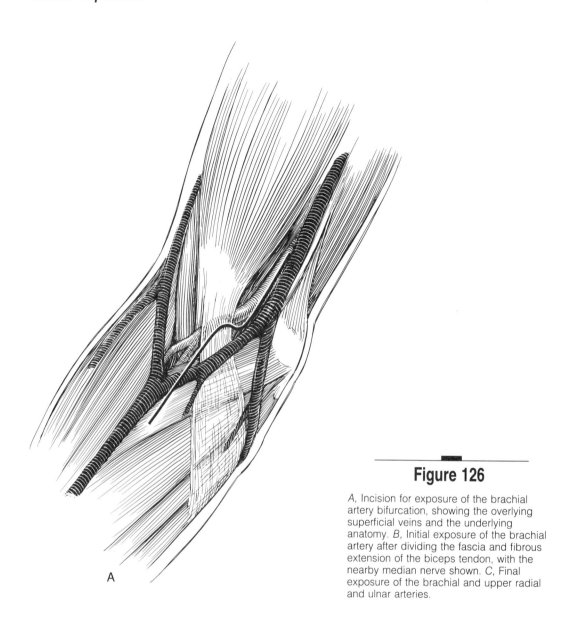

A

Figure 126

A, Incision for exposure of the brachial artery bifurcation, showing the overlying superficial veins and the underlying anatomy. *B,* Initial exposure of the brachial artery after dividing the fascia and fibrous extension of the biceps tendon, with the nearby median nerve shown. *C,* Final exposure of the brachial and upper radial and ulnar arteries.

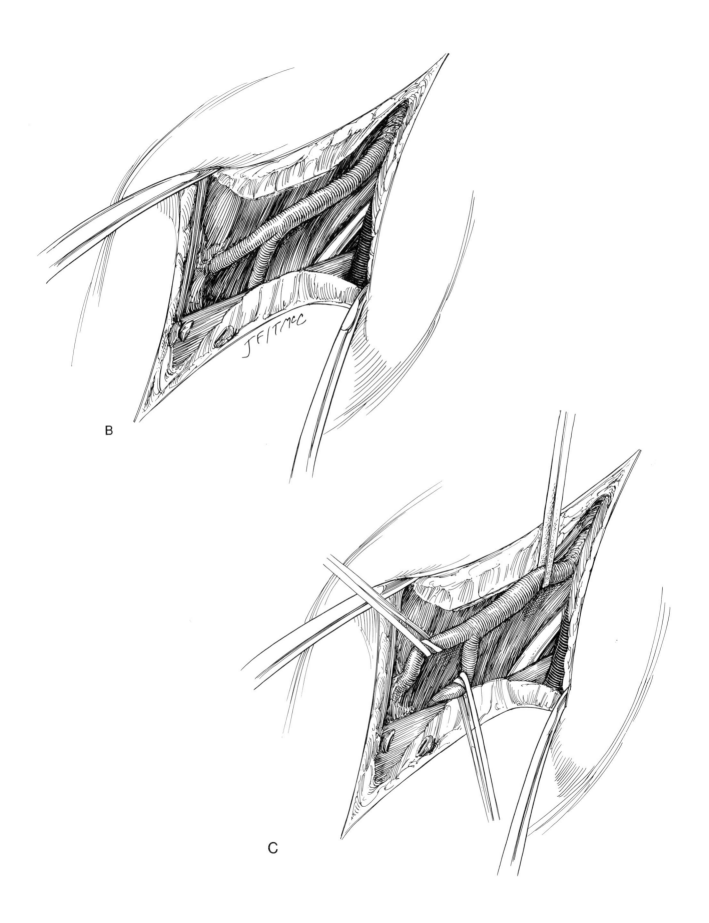

B

C

Vascular Exposures

Exposure of the Distal Radial and Ulnar Arteries at the Wrist. Short longitudinal incisions over these arteries are usually placed for angioaccess (cannulation or creation of arteriovenous fistulas). Because they are usually patent and palpable in these situations, incision placement is not usually a problem. Figure 127 shows both vessels exposed, demonstrating relationships to nearby structures.

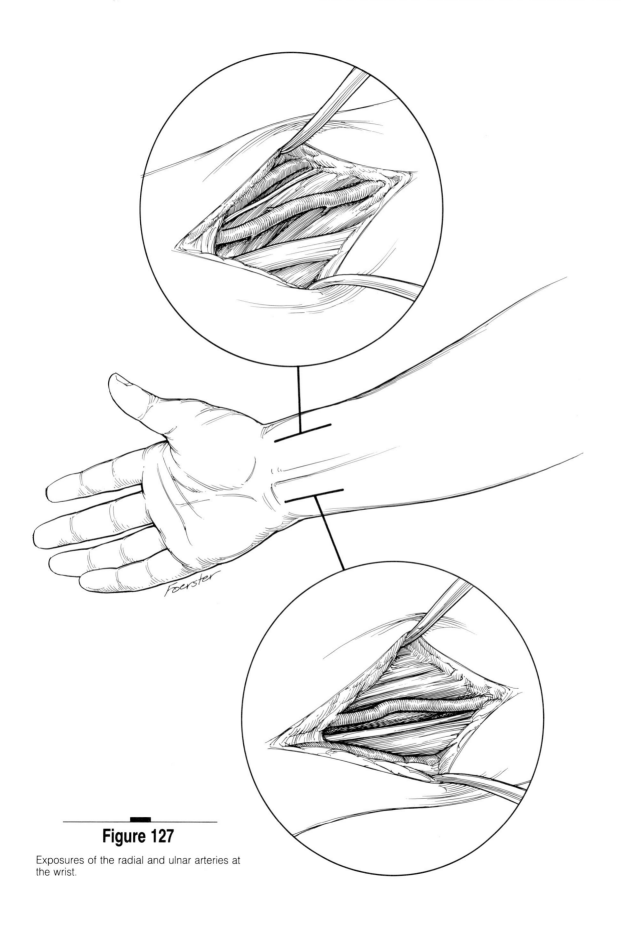

Figure 127

Exposures of the radial and ulnar arteries at
the wrist.

INDEX

Note: Page numbers in *italics* refer to illustrations.

Forceps, jewelers, 6, *9*
    vascular, 4, *5*

Gastrocnemius muscle, in posterior approach to popliteal vessels, 140, *141–142*
Gastroduodenal artery, exposure of, 218, *219–221*
Gerota's fascia, in aortic exposure, 198, *199*
Glossopharyngeal nerve, in carotid artery exposure, 242, *243*
Gonadal vessels, in thoracoabdominal aortic exposure, 232
Gore-Tex PTFE graft, 54, *57*
Graft. See also *Autograft.*
    cephalic vein, 71
    Dacron, in end-to-side anastomosis, 54, *57*
        in patch angioplasty, 32
    Gore-Tex PTFE, 54, *57*
    history of, 2–3, 70–71
    in end-to-side anastomosis, 48, *49–51*, 54, *57*
        rounding or squaring tip of, 58, *59*
        suturing in, with limited mobility of vessel or graft, 58, *61*, 62, *63*
    infected, permanent vascular interruption techniques in, 24
    polytetrafluoroethylene, in end-to-side anastomosis, 54, *57*
    saphenous vein, 70
Gregory clamp, 6, *9*

Heifitz clips, 6, *9*
Hemostasis. See also *Exposure, and control.*
    permanent, 24, *26*, *27*
    temporary, 2, 28
Heparin, general considerations for, 28–29
    in vein harvest, 74
    protamine sulfate and, 29
Hepatic artery, exposure of, 218, *219–221*
    mesenteric, superior, exposure of, *188–193*, *205*, *207*, 210–211, 216–217, *216–217*
Heterograft. See also *Graft.*
    history of, 2–3, 70
History, of vascular surgery, 2–3
Homograft. See also *Graft.*
    arterial, 70
    history of, 2–3, 70–71
    saphenous vein, 70
Hydragrip clamp, 6, *8*
Hypogastric artery, in aortic exposure, 180–181, *180–183*
Hypoglossal nerve, in carotid artery exposure, 238, *239–241*, 242

Iliac artery, circumferential control of, 22, *22–23*, 24, *25*
    in aortic exposure, 177, *178–185*, 180–181, 184, 186. See also *Aorta, exposure of, iliac arteries in.*
    thoracoabdominal, 232
    interruption techniques for, 24, *25–27*
Instrument(s). See also names of specific instruments.
    basic, 4, *5*, 6, *7–9*, *8*

Instrument(s) *(Continued)*
    valvulotomy, 76, *79–80*
Intubation, nasotracheal, in high internal carotid artery exposure, 242
Ischemia, mesenteric, 216–217, *216–217*

Jeweler's forceps, 6, *9*
Jugular vein, in carotid artery exposure, 238, *239–241*
    in supraclavicular exposure of subclavian artery, 244, 248, *248*, *249*

Kidney, in retroperitoneal approach to aortic exposure, 198, *198–201*, 202, *205*, 206, *207*
    in thoracoabdominal aortic exposure, 230, 232
Kocher maneuver, *220*

Lidocaine, in carotid artery exposure, 238, *241*
Lymphatics, in exposure of lower extremities, 120, *122–123*

Mandible, in high internal carotid artery exposure, 242, *243*
Maxilla, in high internal carotid artery exposure, 242, *243*
Mesenteric artery, in thoracoabdominal aortic exposure, 232
    superior, exposure of, *188–193*, *205*, *207*, 210–211, 216–217, *216–217*
Metzenbaum scissors, 4, *5*, 11, *11*, 12
Microvascular surgery, 6
Minivascular surgery, 6, *9*
Muscle(s), digastric, in high internal carotid artery exposure, *243*
    gastrocnemius, in posterior approach to popliteal vessels, 140, *141–142*
    pectoralis, in infraclavicular exposure, 250, *252*
    platysma, in supraclavicular exposure of subclavian artery, 244, *246–247*
    sartorius, in exposure of distal profunda femoris, *114*, 124–125, *128*
        in medial exposure of above-knee popliteal artery, *137*
    sternocleidomastoid, in carotid artery exposure, 237, 238, *239–241*
        in supraclavicular exposure of subclavian artery, 244, *246–247*
    stylohyoid, in carotid artery exposure, *243*
    subclavius, in infraclavicular exposure, 251

Nasotracheal intubation, in carotid artery exposure, 242
NAVEL, 120
Needle, selection of, 8
Needle holder, 4, *5*
    Castroviejo, 6, *9*
Nerve(s), accessory, in carotid artery exposure, 242

ISBN 0-7216-2956-3